Choosing Waterbirth

"A spiritual breath of fresh air reflecting heartfelt practical tools during pregnancy, labor, birth, and parenting. An inspirational gift to help women remember what's too often forgotten: our bodies and our babies know how."

—Judith E. Halek, director of Birth Balance, a waterbirth center in New York

"Lakshmi graciously creates a way of birthing that is supported by nature and surrounded by love. After floating through ***Choosing Waterbirth***, I feel as if I have been reborn."

—Nischala Joy Devi, author of *The Healing Path of Yoga*

Choosing Waterbirth

reclaiming the sacred power of birth

Lakshmi Bertram

for the evolving human spirit
HAMPTON ROADS
PUBLISHING COMPANY, INC.

Cover design by Grace Pedalino
Cover art by Frank Riccio
Photos by Stephanie Gross

For information write:

Hampton Roads Publishing Company, Inc.
1125 Stoney Ridge Road
Charlottesville, VA 22902

Or call: 804-296-2772
FAX: 804-296-5096
e-mail: hrpc@hrpub.com
Web site: www.hrpub.com

If you are unable to order this book from your local bookseller, you may order directly from the publisher. Call 1-800-766-8009, toll-free.

Library of Congress Catalog Card Number: 99-95406

ISBN 1-57174-152-6

10 9 8 7 6 5 4 3 2 1

Printed on acid-free paper in Canada

Dedication

This book is lovingly dedicated to my children,

Sampath, Nataraja, Rani, Madhuri, and Lalita,

without whom I would not be a mother.

And to all the sweet babies of the world

who bring us love and joy unbounded.

Acknowledgements

I would like to thank my most Beloved Sri Gurudev, Sri Swami Satchidananda, for being the guiding light in my life, for protecting me from harm, and for encouraging me always to be my highest Self.

Thanks to my husband, Nilakantan, for being my partner through thick and thin, for being there for me whenever I need him, for loving me and being my funny companion, and for having the original idea that got me started on this project in the first place.

A most hearty thanks to my children for teaching me about love and joy, selflessness and patience; to my mother for sweet lullabies and card games and popcorn; to my father for cowboy songs and Candan Deseme; to each one of my beautiful sisters, and my equally beautiful brother, for their unrivaled encouragement and support; and to my extended family, the Yogaville Community, for all that they have meant to me throughout my life.

Thanks to Rivers Cuomo for wading through a deluge of letters—and for loving them; to Pat Thornton for the new author package and for saying, "Hey, you should write a book on waterbirth"; to Prakash Shakti for first believing in me and for encouraging me to keep on writing; to Jyothi Caroll for teaching me how to believe in myself; to Ken Eagle Feather for seeing my potential and for being willing to work with the possibilities; and to everyone else who has expressed an interest in my writing, excitement about my book, and enthusiasm for my ideas.

Thanks to Dr. Sandra McLanahan, Janet Balaskas, Judith Halek, Michel Odent, Sheila Kitzinger, Ina May Gaskin, and Barbara Harper for lending their professional support and guidance to this project.

Thanks to Richard Leviton, my editor, for helping me to write *this* book and for showing me very clearly where to go right.

And a very special thanks to Bob Friedman who opted to publish my book even though, as he said, "We don't usually publish this kind of thing"; and thanks to the rest of the people at Hampton Roads Publishing Company who, aside from being wonderful, have become like an extended family to me.

Thanks everyone.

Contents

Part IV—The Celebration and Afterwards

Preface

While reading *Choosing Waterbirth* by Lakshmi Bertram I could not help thinking of a recent comment made by a well-known British professor of obstetrics. He was wondering why there are still women who want to go through the stress and pain of labor at a time when it is possible—thanks to epidurals and drips—to give birth and watch TV at the same time. I could not help thinking also of a recent survey among British women obstetricians: one third of them would prefer not even to try to give birth naturally and would choose to have an elective C-section. I wish these so-called experts in childbirth were given the opportunity to listen to this other category of experts, as exemplified by the author of this book.

Lakshmi writes as a mother. She focuses on the births of her five babies. My role is to enlarge the topic and to hint at those who made different choices and also who gave birth without any precise plan. To do so, I'll just select a significant anecdote.

In the late 1970s an Italian woman from Venice came to our hospital in France to give birth. This woman was a diver and a doctor who specialized in diving medicine. She used to spend two hours a day in water. She was convinced that a birthing pool was, for her, the only possible place to give birth. That is why she traveled here from another country at a time when the idea of a birthing pool had not yet spread out. The day of the birth she spent some minutes in the water, got out of the pool, and finally gave birth on the dry land, like most women.

On the following days she was sharing a double room with a local woman who had previously claimed that all these "tricks" (such as the use of water during labor) were good only for "crazy women coming from far away."

When in hard labor, this same local woman was irresistibly attracted by the water and she eventually entered the birthing pool. She had complete privacy while in the water—having the father present or using a camera was only good for "crazy women coming from far away." There was nobody else around other than an experienced and low-profile midwife. The labor was therefore fast and easy. It did not take long before she reached this particular state of consciousness clearly described by Lakshmi as the time when the mother-to-be is "dropping back into instinct, instead of reason, feeling instead of thinking." In another language, I would say that she had reduced her neocortical control. While in such a state of consciousness she knew that her baby could be born safely under water. She did not get out of the bath until the contractions announcing the placenta began.

These two happy mothers became good friends, overcoming their differing backgrounds and their language barrier. Seemingly their experiences of childbirth were different, but in fact, they had just used different ways to reach the authentic knowledge of this unique short period of time when a woman becomes a mother—the authentic knowledge Lakshmi is so clearly able to express with words.

—Dr. Michel Odent,
author of *Birth Reborn*

Foreword

I highly recommend everyone read this book. It contains wisdom not only for prospective parents, but for all of us. It celebrates a unique approach to birthing, but also paints a vision for the way in which we humans can reconnect to the strength and joy of our intuitive and spiritual selves, living in fullest harmony with nature.

What makes this book especially valuable is that Lakshmi writes from her own experience. She brings much-needed poetic beauty and thoughtful reflection to a pivotal arena of our lives. Especially necessary are patience and tolerance for the varying rhythms of natural childbirth, as she so meaningfully explores. The song of the heart is written here with melodic, meditative awareness.

Power rests in tranquillity. Surrounding yourself with inspiration is always helpful, but is especially influential during pregnancy. This book provides images and suggestions that can help you make your birthing journey a sacred one.

Most people love the water. I run to the ocean whenever I can, hike alongside waterfalls on weekends, and lean back into a warm bath daily. The peacefulness of a serene soak after a tough day has obvious stress-relieving effects. Since eighty percent of illness is stress-related, we need to find ways to address this component, both preventively and therapeutically. Water is a simple, available, inexpensive, and effective antidote to stress.

We now understand that the physical stress of labor and delivery is significantly influenced by the important connection of body and mind, and mind to body. Both mother and baby are affected by tension, worry, or any physical or mental strain. Techniques that can reduce these elements, such as the breathing methods discussed by Lakshmi, can serve to help the mother maintain a state of relaxation beneficial to her own health and that of the child, and help assure a smooth delivery.

Water provides an especially powerful tool to help in this relaxation process. Most women associate bathing with stress-release, and this connection alone can serve to assist them during labor and delivery. The physical benefits of the warm water include directly allowing the muscles to relax. Since tense muscles have higher oxygen requirements, this reduction in their strain helps ensure that optimum blood supply and nutrition can be available for creating balanced hormone release and, thereby, ease of delivery. The hormones associated with stress, such as adrenaline, impair this process.

For the first ten years of my family medical practice I included obstetrics. I loved assisting women to have their babies, and began to use the LeBoyer bathing method, immersing infants in a warm tub of water soon after they were born. I witnessed the joy of these babies' relaxation, as they stretched their cramped limbs with obvious relief and delight.

I had been conventionally trained, where all the women were lying on their backs, feet up in stirrup, the attending doctors joking about other things, treating the birthing mothers as if they had no feelings, and were simply there to be attended to, like dumb animals, or even, considering the humanity of many veterinarians, much worse. Most of the obstetricians were men, with little sympathy and no apparent empathy for what their patients were experiencing. Would *you* want to have even a bowel movement (to say nothing of a baby) lying on your back with your feet up in the air?

My first home delivery completely changed my perspective on birthing's possibilities. Close friends had asked me to help them create a peaceful and natural childbirth. What a wondrous difference, to see the ease and comfort possible when the mother stayed at home, in a cozy setting, delivering in her own bed, in a semi-sitting, semi-squatting position as the process was allowed to unfold at its own pace. I was hooked. The contrast with conventional care was so stunning I became an active home-birth advocate, and offered that option for many of my patients.

We come into this life "trailing clouds of glory," as the poet Wordsworth put it. I believe that we are, at our essence, spiritual beings. We take on a body to learn lessons, and keeping this in mind helps us come through any challenges we may face. At one extraordinary home birth, the electricity in the house went out just as the child's head was crowning, so I had to deliver the baby entirely by feel, in pitch darkness! That particular soul seemed to have wanted to come into this world in the most natural way possible; the lights, which we had placed on a dim setting, came gently back on just a few moments after it was born.

The most urgent question is, of course—about both home births and waterbirthing—are they really safe? Evidence from countries that have organized back-up for home births, such as the Netherlands, indicates that this option can be even more safe in routine births than a hospital delivery, which increases risk for complications and infections. Waterbirthing has thus far also shown itself to be both very safe and effective.

Many hospitals are now offering a more home-like, natural setting for birthing and tubs for labor and delivery. Another feature is birthing centers, which are specialized facilities where only birthing takes place, insuring adequate emergency availability but less risk for infection than in conventional hospitals.

A child's first experiences after birth may affect its entire life framework. Much research has supported the importance of mother-infant bonding, which influences later child-rearing, I.Q., and both physical and emotional health of mother and baby.

The physical and mental comfort of both mother and baby is crucial. We must act to reduce the current one-in-four cesarean section rate in the U.S., which translates to a mother suffering discomfort from the after-effects of surgery for one-in-four newborn babies. Research supports opposition to routine episiotomies and circumcisions—again to reduce unneeded pain.

Lakshmi's book provides inspiration and support for women to learn to turn away from excess interventions, to return to the innate wisdom of the body and its natural resources. Waterbirthing, either in hospital or elsewhere, can provide important comfort and relaxation, reduce the necessity of drugs, and, when necessary, be combined with conventional medicine for the best of both worlds.

You should consider each birthing choice on an individual basis in consultation with your doctor. Lakshmi's instructive and inspiring book can help you create a context in which to make those choices more knowledgeably, to help provide the most protected and at the same time gentle welcome for each new soul on our planet—for the physical, emotional, and spiritual health of us all.

—Sandra Amrita McLanahan, M.D.

Part I

The Theory

chapter 1

Soul Searching

Every woman, when she finds out she is carrying a new life, asks herself a number of difficult and soul-searching questions. "Am I ready for this? Will I be a good mother? Will I be able to do all that will be demanded of me in the years to come?" We all face the same fears and doubts about our ability to create a new life, bring it safely into the world, and raise it successfully.

Probably the most difficult of these questions, and the one most agonized over, concerns the actual birth. "Will I be able to do it? Will I be able to make it through the labor and delivery?" Fears about the intensity of the contractions and of being unable to push the baby out are utmost in the mother's mind, causing anxiety in some and a crippling fear in others.

In today's society, it is no wonder so many women fear birth. Who hasn't seen a birth on film or television where a wailing baby is pulled from a mother who is writhing and screaming in pain and swearing she will never have a baby again? Who hasn't heard the birth horror stories told by women who have gone through the process? Today, birth is commonly viewed as overwhelming and frightening and, because of this, many women no longer see it as a natural occurrence that they have the ability to get through.

For thousands of years, women have been giving birth. As women, our bodies and minds are uniquely adapted to it. When we were created inside the wombs of our mothers, our bodies were already at work giving us this unique ability. Birth is a natural, healthy process that if left up to nature can be one of the greatest and most joyful experiences of our lives.

We trust in nature for so many things: respiration, assimilation, digestion, the beating of our hearts. Without nature, we would immediately die, no oxygen would enter our lungs, no blood would carry this oxygen to the necessary places and all cells would cease to function. Our very ability to exist depends on nature. Yet, somehow we have come to believe that in this one particular area of childbearing, nature has failed and we women no longer have the ability to give birth!

In fact, as many dismayed husbands, taxi drivers, and rescue personnel will tell you, no matter where they are or what is going on around them, when a baby is ready to be born, it is usually born. It may be in the hospital, the taxi, a shopping mall, an elevator, in a tree, as I recently heard on the news of a woman who did this, or it may be at home. When the moment of birth arrives, nature waits for no one. Most births do not actually require doctors or hospitals or fetal monitors or forceps or episiotomies or drugs. Once babies are ready, they arrive and the only other person needed is the mother.

And every mother can give birth naturally. If allowed to follow your natural inclinations, you can labor and birth your baby in your own unique way, relying on your own strength, tuning into an inner knowledge that only you possess.

We all have this ability; it's built into our systems. With the onset of labor, your consciousness will shift and you will become more subconscious in your thinking patterns, dropping back from reason into instinct, from thinking into feeling. In this highly intuitive state, you will know exactly what you want and need to be able to birth your baby. If respected, and given what you instinctually desire, you will very likely be able to give birth without interference, just as you were designed to do. If your instinctual preferences are ignored, however, as they often are in the typical hospital setting, that is when you could need "help" from outside.

Hospitals, while well-intentioned, typically do not allow for this natural process. It was for this reason that I chose to give birth at home. Hospitals, in their narrow, clinical view, tend to expect babies to be born on time, following the averages, and according to a predetermined schedule. They appear to overlook that birth is unpredictable, changing, and flowing like everything else in nature. And that, while there are certain processes that must occur for the baby to be born, there are many variations on how these processes come about and that most of these variations are normal. Because of this view, labor and birth are "managed" and often chemically altered with drugs to ensure that they meet the hospital criteria.

In contrast to the gentleness and consideration I believe childbirth deserves is the typical hospital birth where a laboring woman entering the hospital to deliver her baby is faced with a situation so inconsiderate of her needs, that it can inspire fear and embarrassment in even the most stouthearted.

My first awareness of this inspired an absolute certainty in me that I did not want to have a hospital birth. I wanted freedom of movement and choice. I wanted to be able to do whatever I needed to feel the most comfortable while birthing my baby. I had heard other women's stories of their hospital births, I knew what they had gone through, and the experiences they had had were not the ones I wanted for myself while I birthed my babies.

If I birthed in the hospital, most likely during labor, I would be strapped immobile to a bed, an IV line in my arm, a monitor around my abdomen. My freedom to move taken from me, I would not be able to walk around to enlist the help of gravity, not be able to squat to shorten the birth canal, not be allowed to stretch, bend, or do any movement at all that would help ease or shorten my labor. I would not be allowed to eat or drink after the onset of labor. Which made me wonder: where would I get energy for the labor and pushing the baby out? During this time when in a natural labor a woman feels a powerful urge to bear down, in the hospital scenario, I was likely to feel exhausted and disheartened.

If I had pain-reducing drugs administered during labor, my pushing ability could be diminished even further, which meant I could also expect to spend hours trying to get my baby out. I would almost certainly be given an episiotomy, which is a surgical cut in the wall of the perineum to make the birth canal bigger. There was a good chance if I went beyond a set time limit, a vacuum or forceps would be used to try to pull the baby out. And I would have a twenty-five percent chance of having a C-section in which my baby would be "born" by being pulled out of me through a surgical incision in my abdomen.

In addition to this, by having to cater to the hospital set-up and the birthing personnel—doctors, nurses, anesthesiologists—this most natural, private, and intimate of moments would become a public affair. Like many women, with so many people around, watching and scrutinizing me, I knew I would feel an incredible pressure to perform, to be "good" at this birthing thing, as if there were a wrong way for me to birth my baby.

The twenty-hour, extremely painful labor brings about just as real a baby as the very quick, two-hour labor does. Both births are equal in the fact that the final result is the same, yet it is often the two-hour birthing woman who is considered the "good birthing" mother and the twenty-hour mother who is deemed deficient. This seemed to be an unfair misconception to me. Obviously the woman who labors longer and harder deserves at least a little more commendation for all her effort. What she usually gets is condemnation.

I did not want this commonly accepted belief that birth should be a certain way to tarnish my experiences of giving birth. Whether I labored for two hours or twenty, I wanted total acceptance and support from all the people around me.

Once my baby was born, there would be a whole new set of concerns. After nine months of waiting and counting the days, once the baby was finally here, I did not want it immediately whisked away. I wanted a chance to get to know the baby I had carried, time to lovingly welcome it to the world, while I held against my breast this whole, new person that I had created. I knew it was common practice in the hospital for the baby to be taken soon after the birth to be checked over, cleaned up, and weighed. To me, all this seemed secondary to taking the time to get to know my baby.

When viewed as a whole, a hospital birth seemed to offer so little. In exchange for "safety," I would be sacrificing consideration and respect. In exchange for a doctor's knowledge, I would be giving up my own inner guidance. In exchange for pain-reduction, I would be giving up freedom and power.

I knew birth was natural and did not need to be feared. I knew as a woman I was capable of giving birth.

I was right.

Into this careful consideration, water labor and delivery were introduced. Keeping with the empowerment and freedom of a natural birth, it brought the added benefit of making labor shorter and less painful. Being safe for the mother because there are no drugs in her system and safe for the baby because a baby will not breathe until its face hits the air, waterbirth was also effective and had no negative side effects. Through waterbirth, I could have pain-reduction while retaining intuitive freedom. Nothing had to be exchanged for the benefits; none of my ideals had to be sacrificed.

Five births later, I can honestly say that all of my experiences were wonderful and fulfilling. Five births later, I can tell you that your birth experiences can be, too.

chapter 2

Nature's Lesson

My first awareness of birth as a natural experience came to me at a very young age. Not, as might be expected, from the stories told by well-meaning aunts and grandmothers, nor from the obvious example of my own mother who had six children. My awareness came from first-hand experience, powerful and more far-reaching than any story. It came from the four-legged friends of mine, the horses, whom I valued at the age of five more than any of my human friends.

Living on my grandparents' horse ranch with my mother and father and my three sisters, I was third down the list of four girls and I was quiet, a dreamer. By the time I was three, I was spending more time in the pasture than in the house. I don't know how old I was when I first began to climb through the gate to mingle with the great beasts on the other side. But I feel quite certain the event nearly gave my mother a heart attack and I feel equally certain she and my father did their best to keep me from venturing in with the horses again. After all, these animals weren't puppies; they were thousand-pound thoroughbred mares. One wrong move, accidental or otherwise, and I would have been sent very quickly to the "great beyond." However, two things soon became apparent, and these allowed me to have a childhood I can never forget.

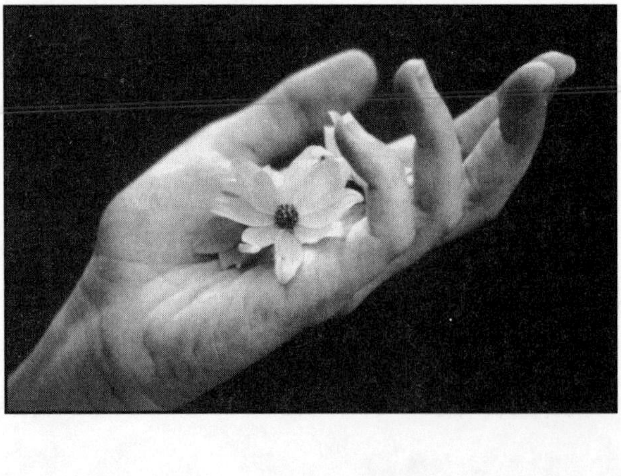

First, there was no way to keep me out of there;

any time I was left on my own, I headed straight for the pasture. Second, the mares took a liking to me, treating me with gentleness and care as if I was one of their own, only considerably smaller. I spent untold hours with the mares, following them through the pasture, wandering in and out of their legs, sleeping in their feed bins. I grew to love them with a passion that is still with me today.

I had one particular favorite. Her name was Rosy May. She was a wide-girthed, gentle quarter horse mare with a beautiful strawberry roan coat and a black mane and tail. I loved her more than any of the others and was rewarded in turn by her total acceptance of me. She would stand perfectly still while I sat leaning against her front legs, singing to her in my off-key voice. Rosy May would allow me to climb on her back when she was resting on her side. When she stood up, I clung to her like a burr and thus spent many hours of my early childhood on horseback.

My mother tells a story about me (much to my adult embarrassment) of how she found me on Rosy May's back one evening, sitting unconcerned, as something wet streamed down the mare's sides. With some amusement she realized the wet streaks were pee. Apparently I was not even willing to get off the horse's back in order to use the bathroom. My mother also tells of looking out her kitchen window and seeing me asleep on the horse's broad back, the gentle giant unmoving while I slept the afternoon away.

These powerful and beautiful creatures were my life and, for a time, I half believed myself to be one of them. Many were brood mares, and each spring would bring the promise of a dozen new foals on the ranch. Next to Rosy May, the foals were the closest to my heart, and I would wait with suppressed excitement for the birthing season. . . .

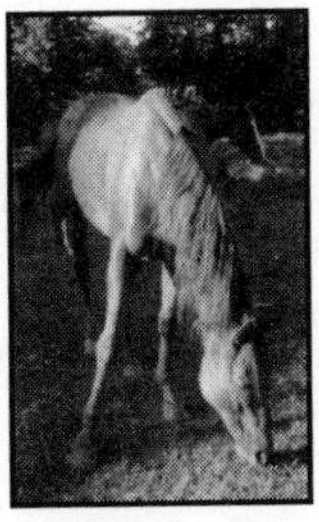

It is 4:00 A.M. on a cold spring morning. A gentle shake awakens me.

"Lakshmi, come on. It's time."

I open my eyes and look into my mother's face leaning over me.

"Hurry!" she whispers. "Or you'll miss it."

Shaking the sleep from my head, I spring from the bed feeling a burst of excitement. Still in my pajamas, I follow her through the quiet house. We pause at the back door to pull on our coats. Then, stepping out into the brisk predawn air, we hurry across the patio towards our destination.

Maybe at that time my sisters are there too, I don't know, I can't remember, because all my attention centers on the dim light coming from the cracks in the side of the barn.

Thwump! A collapsing sound comes from the barn as the mare lies down.

"She's dropped!" Mom smiles at me excitedly. "Quickly, now. Come quietly. We don't want to frighten her."

I scramble up the side of the barn to the window opening, trying to be quiet, even in my haste. Peering into the eerie semi-darkness made red by a heat lamp suspended from the ceiling, I see the mare. She lies dark against the straw, her sides heaving, her gaze turned inwards. She breathes long slow breaths, deeply relaxing. She doesn't appear concerned or frightened by what she is doing, even when the muscles of her abdomen tighten with the next contraction. I watch wide-eyed and silent as she begins to breathe quicker, almost panting through the peak of the contraction; then as it slides away, forgotten, she takes deep, soothing breaths, releasing her tension, allowing her strength to return for the next one.

The mare labors naturally in the rhythm of birth. Breathing, allowing each contraction to do its job, relaxing completely in between to keep up her strength. Soon a subtle shift begins. Now, during the height of each contraction, the mare holds her breath and engages her abdominal muscles to begin the job of pushing her little passenger out into the world. The contractions become more intense and before long, the forelegs appear, covered in the pink amniotic sac. On the next push, a head appears, followed soon after by the foal. It wriggles, tearing the sac, and I get my first glimpse of the new arrival.

Soaking wet, its hair plastered to its head, making its already large ears appear even bigger, the foal is not much to look at. But as the wide black eyes turn my way, I know that I've never seen anything as beautiful.

The new mother sits up straight and cranes her head around to examine the foal. Her eyes are bright and curious as she nuzzles her baby; all the pain of labor is forgotten in the magic moment of birth. I sigh, resting my chin on my arms, filled with awe by the miracle I have witnessed.

To me, all this seems normal, business as usual. There were no doctors, no bright lamps, no fetal monitors or forceps, and the mother felt safe and comfortable in her familiar surroundings with no need for painkillers. Long before I had ever heard of "natural birth," I had witnessed it many times in the dimly lit interior of a foaling shed and from these experiences came the absolute belief that this is the way birth was meant to be.

Many years later, when I received the news, via a home pregnancy test, that I was to have a baby, I knew that I wanted to do it at home without interference or drugs. I wanted to do it naturally, in a dimly lit room with warmth and silence surrounding me, just as I had seen it done so often by the "playmates" of my childhood, the mares.

chapter 3

A Challenging Reality

Deciding to give birth naturally was one thing; having to seriously consider going through all that labor without painkillers was another thing entirely.

Birth may be beautiful, but it is also challenging. It is to women what a coming of age ceremony might be to men. It is a time when we must reach deep inside ourselves to find a strength we didn't know we possessed until the moment comes and it is needed. During this time, nothing outside of us can help; no person and no thing can birth our babies for us. It is our bodies that must open up to allow these babies to be born, and our minds that must accept the pain caused by their births. Midwives and doctors, husbands and friends may offer us support and guidance, but it is we who must actually go through the process.

Knowing this it was with some trepidation and a lot of determination that I decided to birth my baby, naturally, at home.

I began reading everything I could about the process of labor and birth, educating myself in the hope of relieving some of the anxiety I was feeling. But there were few books on the subject that could tell me what I wanted to know. Many of them addressed the physical process of labor and delivery in great detail, but fell short of providing me with any practical advice, or even information, about having my baby naturally, at home. Living in a rural community, forty-five miles from the nearest big town, neither did I have access to Lamaze, or any other birth organization or childbirth education class that could offer support and encouragement.

What I did have was a firm belief in natural birth that was shared and supported by my immediate family and also the spiritual community in which I lived. This belief and support is what caused me to choose home birth, but it was one particular book, *Spiritual Midwifery*, that gave me what I needed to feel truly comfortable with that decision.

The book, written by Ina May Gaskin, who was the primary midwife in the spiritual community called "The Farm" in Tennessee where the natural births depicted in the book were taking place, appealed to me because it was so in line with what I already believed. *Spiritual Midwifery* filled in the missing link. I already had the belief; *Spiritual Midwifery* provided the practical advice. From this book I learned that knowledge does have an influence over matter, that by knowing my cervix was opening with each contraction, I could not only help myself to be more accepting of the pain, but could actually help my cervix to open faster. This was very encouraging. It made me feel that I would not have to suffer helplessly, but could actually play an active role in giving birth to my babies. It made me feel more comfortable with my choice and allowed me the mental freedom to relax and enjoy my pregnancy.

My first pregnancy went beautifully. I am graced to be one of those few lucky women who love being pregnant. All the good things that are *supposed* to happen during pregnancy happened to me. I got just the right amount of morning sickness, enough to make me feel like a pregnant woman, but not enough to prevent me from enjoying the experience. I was content with my changing body and suffused with energy and light. I was energetic and serene and had never before felt so complete.

Pregnancy was for me the ultimate feminine experience, and I spent those nine months marveling at being able to create a child. I would look in my many birthing books to see in what stage of growth the baby was, and as the pregnancy progressed and the due date drew nearer, my anxiety about giving birth began to fade, replaced by a keen eagerness to see this developing person.

By the time the ninth month came, there was only one thing left that was bothering me. One of the childbirth preparation exercises I learned from my reading—that was also suggested by my midwife—was the use of visual imagery as preparation for the birth. To do this, you settle into a comfortable position, usually in a relaxed sitting or lying down position, and picture yourself giving birth.

All my life I had done similar visualization practices in yoga, so initially this exercise was easy for me. I would relax, watch my breathing and feel the tension leave me, and then I would begin my visualization. Everything would begin all right. I would picture myself relaxed and happy in my house, feeling my excitement and anticipation of the event. I would see myself going through the labor, breathing with each contraction, handling them as they grew more intense. I visualized myself in transition, which, as the cervix opens to the full ten centimeters, is often the most difficult time of the birth—here, I would be relaxed, breathing, succeeding. However, when I came to the pushing stage, my visualization would stop. I could not see a laboring position that I felt would be good for me, I could not picture myself in the pushing stage, and I could not visualize the baby being born at all. Try as I might, I could not visualize the birth.

One week before I was due, Mary Carmichael, who was to be my midwife, introduced me to the idea of giving birth in water. I had never heard of it before, but I was intrigued, attracted by the idea of an entirely natural supplement to home birth that offered pain-reduction for me and a gentler entry for my baby.

Though there was very little information about waterbirth available at the time, Mary, who had been interested in waterbirth for a couple of years, had recently attended a lecture given by Michael Rosenthal and Michel O'Dent, two pioneers of waterbirth, at the University of Virginia. In addition to this I was able to watch a video called *Water Baby: Experiences of*

Water Birth, produced by Karil Daniels of Point of View Productions. In this video, three couples gave birth to their babies in water. It was amazing, like the answer to a prayer, to see this video.

Laboring and delivering in water was supposed to be less painful. The women in the video looked strong and confident. It was supposed to be gentler for the baby. The babies looked serene and otherworldly, floating to the surface to draw their first breaths as their faces came into contact with the air, and then quietly awakening to the world. Seeing them, I decided that I wanted to birth my babies in the same way.

That same week Nilakantan, my husband, and I went to our local feed store and purchased an eighty-gallon, fiberglass horse and cattle trough that was to be our birthing tub. As I looked down into the three-foot deep black tub, knowing I would soon be giving birth in it, I was finally able to complete the visualization of my birth.

The next week, after a textbook labor, I gave birth to my first water baby, Sampath Moses. I will never forget the sensation I felt as I lowered myself into the water. Immediately, I was almost weightless and the unbearable pressure that had felt like a tight band across the bottom of my abdomen was gone. I sighed, sinking deeper into the water, completely relaxing. As the next contraction came, I found I could handle it better, breathing deeply through it; as it passed, it seemed that every spare muscle in my body turned to jelly and all the tension dissolved into the warmth of the water. Soon I was falling asleep between contractions, drifting away somewhere, forgetting even that I was in labor.

Like the answer to a prayer, waterbirth met my criteria about giving birth naturally in the most gentle and caring way I could. Afterwards, I felt a true sense of accomplishment, as if I had done something huge and amazing. And so I had. I had accomplished my goal of bringing a child into this world in a way that recognized and honored what an amazingly tough event it is to be born and what a fantastic and difficult thing it is to give birth. I think this is what every birth is meant to be: an experience that leaves a woman feeling accomplished and strong, a child feeling loved and secure. Birthing is a rite of passage for woman and baby. It is not simply about bringing a body out of a body, but about bringing a soul from a soul.

chapter 4

Why Water?

Most people are drawn to water. After a hard day's work, few things feel better than a soak in the tub. Likewise, in the midst of the summer months, few things are as refreshing as a cool swim. Water soothes, relaxes, and rejuvenates, providing an easy way to unwind and let go of the tensions built up during the day.

During pregnancy, water becomes even more desirable. As the pregnancy progresses and your body grows heavier and more unwieldy, total immersion may be the only time you feel relief from the constant pressure of the growing fetus on your lower back and pelvic region. Soaking in the tub at this time can feel so good, you may never wish to get out.

It is partly because of this that the first recorded waterbirth came about.

In 1805 in a small village in France, a woman labored long and hard to birth her baby. After two days, she was physically and mentally exhausted. As hydrotherapy was common in 1800s France, the attending doctor suggested the use of a bath. I know how she must have felt sinking into that water. To her, it must have seemed like the only reprieve from a nightmare. The doctor and others looked on, unsuspecting of the rapid changes that were happening inside her body. What they did notice was the almost immediate relaxation that being in the water provided, causing her to have a peaceful, composed, expression. Only a quarter of an hour later, pushing contractions began and the woman remained in the water, where her baby was born. Even though her labor had been lengthy and difficult, after their waterbirth, mother and baby were reported as being in good health, consistent with a normal labor and delivery.

Midwives the world over have often used water in various forms during labor and birth. Hot showers and hot towels are used to ease lower back pain during the contractions, hot compresses are applied to the highly elastic tissue called the perineum next to the vaginal opening to help it to soften and stretch, and cool cloths are laid across the back of the neck and on the forehead to sooth and relax. The natural soothing properties of water for labor and birth have long been noted, but it was only fairly recently that actual delivery of the infant into water was used.

In the early 1960s, Igor Charkovsky pioneered the use of water for labor and delivery in the former Soviet Union. Later in the 1980s, Michel O'Dent spearheaded the movement in France, and in Europe. Since then waterbirth has migrated to many other countries, including the U.S., and it has been estimated that nearly 25,000 women have given birth in water in the U.S. since 1981.

This growth happened even though the medical establishment has not especially accepted the waterbirthing method; even though there are a very limited number of qualified practitioners who attend waterbirths; and even though it is very difficult to acquire a tub. Even with these obstacles, women continue to choose to birth their babies in water. In light of this the question becomes–why? What is it about waterbirth that has so many women making this choice for their births?

chapter 5

The Great Appeal

A universal statement for a woman who has had one waterbirth is that she would "never give birth in any other way." I have found this to be personally true. Having had my first baby in water, I never even considered anything else. The pain was so reduced that in contrast to, "I will never have another baby again!" which is typically uttered after a first baby's birth, I said, as I gazed down at the baby in my arms, "I could do that again, not right away, but in a few years, definitely."

This is a very different statement. It meant that my experience of birth did not leave me feeling helpless, or worn out, or beaten up, or degraded. It meant that I remained feeling capable and confident about my ability to give birth even immediately after the event. This is part of the reason why waterbirth is so appealing. It allows you to view every part of your birth, even the intense parts, as a positive experience.

In addition to this empowerment, laboring and delivering in water has actual, physical advantages.

During childbirth endorphins are released in your body which help you feel less pain. However, anxiety can cause the release of adrenaline, which inhibits the effect of the endorphins. Adrenaline also inhibits the release of oxytocin, the hormone that causes uterine labor contractions, which means feeling anxious and nervous can not only make you feel more pain, but it can also make your contractions less effective.

Getting into a soothing tub of water relaxes you and allows your body's natural endorphins and oxytocin to kick in. Immediately, your contractions are less painful and more effective, which may account for why waterbirths are proving to be consistently shorter than traditional births.

On top of the internal relaxation effect is the topical effect of the warm water. It is supportive and surrounding. It buoys you up and cradles you in its warmth. It allows tight and tired muscles to relax fully, to release their tension and to be rejuvenated for the next contraction. The water also acts topically to soften the tissues of the perineum, making episotomies much less necessary, and causing fewer, and less severe, tears.

Alternately, epidurals, the injection of a local anesthetic into your lower spine to provide numbness from your lower back down, while touted as safe, effective pain-relievers, can cause a host of problems. If you have an epidural, you are more likely to have a forcep or vacuum delivery, where your baby is pulled from the birth canal with metal tongs or with a suction cup attached to his head. There is a greater risk of the fetal heart rate slowing down from lack of oxygen because your blood pressure has fallen way down, your pushing stage is likely to be considerably longer, and you are twice as likely to have a cesarean section.

In contrast, when a person is immersed in a tub of warm water, the blood flow actually increases, providing more oxygenated blood for both you and your baby, which may be another part of the reason that the contractions appear to be even more effective in water. Waterbirths are also notably shorter in both the dilation stage when the cervix is opening to the full ten centimeters, and in the pushing stage when the baby is pushed down through the birth canal and out. And there are none of the long-term negative side effects associated with epidurals, such as backaches, migraines, neck pain, or local numbness.

Viewed as a whole, it is no mystery why waterbirth is growing so rapidly in popularity. It offers so many benefits—less pain, shorter labors, no negative side effects for the mother, all within keeping to the ideal of a natural birth–that *not* choosing a waterbirth is the greater mystery.

chapter 6

First Impressions

Another advantage of waterbirth is how it alters the baby's experience of being born. Consider for a moment what a baby goes through on its way into the world. What a difficult thing it is to be born, being squeezed and molded and then drawing a first breath. Probably the most risky and harrowing journey of our lives, it is in fact, our first physical experience. Up to that point, we were warmly and safely encased in water. All our needs were met as we floated weightlessly, listening to the steady rhythm of our mother's heart. When the moment of birth came, all that changed. We had to breathe immediately or we would die; we had to cry out for food and comfort; we had to hold our own against the unfamiliar force of gravity. Coming into this world, we were immediately challenged and our first impressions of it were of the fight and struggle to survive.

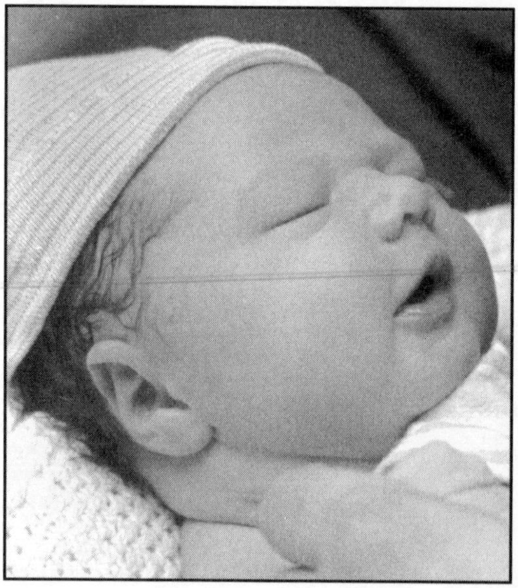

Consider what it's like to be so new and bewildered. All your experiences to date are of being warm and cared for. Imagine the shock of the cold air. It is at this moment that a new baby breathes, taking its first searing breath as its lungs expand and air rushes in. Imagine how that must feel. From the cocoon of the womb, we squeezed down the birth canal, and the first thing we are met with is cold air.

Our next experience is of bright lights. New eyes that have only seen the rosy glow of the sun through the pregnant mother's belly, now open and are blinded by lights. Then there is the noise, the loud, unmuffled, snapping of orders, the issuing of commands; even the happy noises of rejoicing are piercing to the new baby's ears.

Confronted with these realities, babies screw their eyes shut and, opening their mouths to exhale their first breath, they wail. So much fear and pain is heard in that first cry. It is the sound of anguish, the sound our hearts make when everything that we have loved and known has been taken from us. Babies feel this way at birth and they cry out for what they have lost, the warmth and security of the womb and the closeness of their mother. They cry because they are bewildered and scared and because they have no other way of letting us know that they do not understand or like what is happening to them. Nothing touches or melts the heart more than this.

Yet how is their plaintive cry met? Once born, they are whisked away, carried to a hard metal scale, wrapped in a cotton blanket (surely an unfamiliar sensation for them) and laid there to be weighed. Silver nitrate is dropped into their eyes to "burn" off the film that covers them, a film that, having protected the eyes from infection in the womb, is now considered a risk factor for infection. Their limbs are checked, stretched for their ability to move. Finally, the babies are "cleaned up" and eventually returned to their mothers.

Hearing her soothing, familiar voice, feeling the touch of her skin, nonetheless the first impression has been made and the baby soon settles into a suspicious watchfulness.

There is a saying in India, "What is made in the cradle, goes to the cremation ground." We take with us every experience of our lives and carry them as the backdrop against which we view what happens today.

What happens in those first few moments after birth are important. They are moments when amazing things happen.

A fetus becomes a person. A woman becomes a mother. And in a phenomenon called bonding the new mother and the new baby fall in love with each other for life. These moments can never be remade. If they are interrupted, they are lost forever.

Instead of this chaotic entry, imagine how much better it would be if all babies were born into an environment suited to their innocence and newness, like a room filled with soft lights and music, the same sort of room in which they were made. What if after being born, they were allowed to lay quietly in their mother's arms, bare skin against bare skin, heart beat to heart beat, slowly awakening to this new world? We could do this for our newborns, could give this gift of consideration and thus create a generation of souls who never had to know the anguish of being born.

There is a book called *Birth Without Violence* by Frederick Leboyer. In the first week I was pregnant, I read it and fell in love with its concepts. I was awed and inspired by the care given to newborns, as reported by Leboyer. I fell in love with the babies, their peaceful, dark eyes gazing serenely at me. This book introduced me to what I already knew: babies are miracles. They are tiny celestial beings who have somehow decided to exist within bodies and in whom, if you look deep enough, you can see the secrets of the universe. So they deserve the kindest, gentlest entry into this world we can provide.

Waterbirth has expanded Leboyer's concepts. In a traditional natural birth, coming down the birth canal into the waiting world, a child will meet cold air. Coming out into warm water, a child feels only familiarity. Safe and secure, he does not breathe because he has come from water into water and he finds that the world he has entered is not so different from the world he has left behind. When brought up to the surface, his face meets the air and he breathes at last. Nestled in his mother's arms, he feels the security of her skin, and hears the soothing hum of her voice as she speaks words of wonder and love. He awakens gently in this kind of environment. He opens and unfolds.

I watched this phenomenon with my first baby's birth. He was so quiet and wide-eyed; you could feel his curiosity as he looked around. That moment to me was like no other. I felt as though I were looking into the midnight sky, his little eyes were that vast. I couldn't imagine sacrificing that moment for anything, short of something needed to maintain the baby's life. It was too moving, precious, and wonderful.

This is the benefit of waterbirth for a baby—a kind, loving, and gentle entry into this world.

chapter 7

Waterbirth Explained

Birth is termed waterbirth when the lower portion of the laboring woman is immersed in water during the delivery stage of her labor, allowing her baby to be born directly into the water. Water labor is when a woman remains immersed for the duration of her labor, then exits the tub prior to actual delivery. Both water labor and waterbirth offer advantages for the mother, but only waterbirth offers the advantage of a gentler entry for the baby.

In most cases, regular tap water is used to fill the birthing tub. Early on, salt was added to the water in order to more closely mirror the amniotic fluid, and to add a sanitizing effect. This was found to be unnecessary, and today is no longer common practice. The water temperature is kept at approximately ninety-eight degrees, which is body temperature.

In a waterbirth, it is generally recommended that the laboring woman not enter the tub until her active phase of labor, when her cervix has dilated beyond four centimeters and her contractions are coming regularly. Getting in before this can slow the labor down instead of facilitating it. This is not a hard and fast rule, but a general practice that can be used as a guideline in determining when to begin filling the birthing tub.

Once the woman has entered the tub, she may remain in the water for the duration of her labor or she may get in and out according to her inclination. A woman may exit the tub if her labor slows down even though she is well into the active phase, which sometimes happens. Getting out and walking around or squatting at this time may help to make her contractions stronger or more regular. She will also get out to allow the practitioner to check her cervix for dilation, or to use the bathroom. Some women spontaneously get out of the tub immediately before the baby is born. Other women plan to get out and never do. Rarely will a woman be able to predict exactly how and what she will be feeling when the moment of birth comes. Planning for both these possibilities is a good idea.

Fathers or other birth helpers may also want to get in the tub. Whether or not you are interested in doing this is something to consider when you are selecting a tub, which I will go into later in this chapter in greater detail. If the father or birth helper is planning to get into the tub with you, they should shower or bathe first. There have been no known incidences of infection in babies born in water to date, but it never hurts to be careful.

Once the baby is born, either the mother, the father, or the birth attendant will bring the baby up to the surface to breathe. It is not necessary to rush the baby to the surface once it has been born. It will still be receiving oxygen from the mother as long as there is blood flowing through the umbilical cord (this can be felt as a rhythmic pulsing when the cord is held between the thumb and forefinger), but you do want to bring the baby up fairly quickly. There have been cases where a baby was kept under water for up to fifteen minutes, while the umbilical cord was still pulsing, with no negative effects. This has been the exception, not the rule. The general consensus is that the baby should be brought immediately to the surface once it has been born, gently lifted and placed on the mother's chest.

After the birth, the mother and baby may remain in the water for as long as they like. This is nice, as the babies seem to enjoy stretching out and relaxing in the wider space.

The placenta, or afterbirth, which will come out anywhere from a few minutes to a half an hour after the baby is born, can either be birthed directly into the water, or into a container while the woman remains standing in the water, or the woman may exit the tub first and birth the placenta once she is out. This is simply a matter of preference.

chapter 8

Making it Happen

Any woman having a normal, healthy pregnancy and not considered a high risk is a good candidate for waterbirth. Abnormal conditions such as prematurity, which results when true labor begins before the thirty-seventh week; abnormal presentations such as a footling breech where the baby's foot is presenting first; and complications with the placenta, or with the delivery itself, which require medical intervention—these are a few of the conditions that contraindicate water labor and waterbirth. Disease or illness of the mother, specific to or independent of her pregnancy, or of the baby, which require careful medical supervision, also contraindicate waterbirth.

If your pregnancy has progressed normally and healthily and you decide that waterbirth is for you, you will be happy to know it is becoming much easier to locate a practitioner and to secure a tub. There are currently over 600 practicing doctors, nurses, midwives, and nurse-midwives worldwide who are qualified to help you with your waterbirth. To find out who attends waterbirths in your area, contact Karil Daniels (Point of View Productions, 2477 Folsom Street, San Francisco, CA 94110, phone: 415-821-0435, e-mail: karil@well.com). She keeps a resource list of all the people who attend waterbirths in the U.S. and abroad. She will charge you a minimal fee for either the entire list, or to search for someone in your area.

Home waterbirths are still much more accessible than birth center or hospital waterbirths as the home birth community has been actively implementing the use of tubs of water for labor and delivery. However, new birth centers are cropping up all over, and even a few hospitals are starting to provide tubs for women to labor in, though they still balk at actual delivery in a tub.

If having immediate medical support close at hand is important to you, you may find that you have to travel to make your dream of waterbirth a reality. I gave birth to my first four children at home, forty-five miles from the nearest hospital. All four pregnancies had been healthy and without complications so I felt comfortable with my decision. During the early part of my fifth pregnancy, complications arose which, though not serious, were worrisome enough for me to opt to deliver my baby in a birth center where I knew medical assistance was immediately available should I, or my baby, need it.

I was fortunate in having a birth center fifty miles from where I live, which meant I only had to travel during labor, but did not have to stay in the town until the baby was born. Other women I know have left their homes, and in some cases, their countries in order to be able to give birth in water. Consult Karil Daniel's list to find out where the nearest birth center or hospital offering waterbirth is. Once you have that information, you can decide whether or not having a waterbirth is important enough to you to travel for the birth.

If you choose to birth at home, it will be easier to implement, but will still present some challenges. The first will be finding an experienced practitioner to be present at your birth. There is no substitute for a good, qualified practitioner, as she can spot trouble before it becomes serious. Unfortunately, midwifery is still outlawed in some states. If you live in one of these states, travel may again have to be part of your agenda.

Another thing to remember when considering where and how you will birth your baby is that birth is unpredictable. Medical knowledge that is used to screen out abnormalities, coupled with good prenatal care, has allowed for a giant leap in making birth safer for mother and baby. But birth still carries some risk. Having your baby at home does not specifically put you or your baby at greater risk. The infant mortality rates remain the same, or are slightly lower for a planned home birth than a hospital birth. However, if you are in the hospital, and an emergency should arise, the facilities are immediately available to cope with the problem.

Your second challenge when planning a home birth is securing a suitable tub, which, again, is not as difficult as it was eleven years ago when I had my first baby. We got around our tub difficulty by going to the local feed store and trying out the watering troughs until we found one that would work. Providing good depth at three and a half feet deep, with plenty of room at two and a half feet wide and five and a half feet long, it was not the most aesthetically pleasing tub, but it did do the trick. Being made of fiberglass, our tub also had insulation value, which was important in trying to keep the water temperature constant.

You can find tubs on-line both for sale and to rent at Aquadoula, P.O. Box 1132, 110 9th Ave. S., Edmonds, WA 98020; website: www.aquadoula.com; phone: 888-217-2229; e-mail: waterbirth@aquadoula.com. To rent a tub will cost a couple hundred dollars; to purchase it will cost around a thousand dollars.

It is a good idea to check out what actual birthing tubs are available, but you should not limit yourself to only that. Waterbirth, like all birth, allows for a lot of variation. I know of women who have given birth in bathtubs, kiddy pools, portable spas, traditional Jacuzzi tubs, tubs specially made for birthing, and even in the warm waters of the ocean and the much cooler waters of the Black Sea. So long as the tub you select is deep enough to cover your abdomen and roomy enough for you and whomever you may wish to have with you to stretch out and move around in, you should be able to enjoy the benefits of laboring and delivering in water. Your tub should be clean, and preferably not have been used for anything else, with the exceptions being a bath or Jacuzzi tub, which can be thoroughly cleaned prior to the birth.

Where you put your tub is also an important consideration. It is not often that you will have eighty or a hundred gallons of water all in one place. Before you decide where to put your tub, you will have to check to see which part of your flooring will support its weight. Prior to our first baby's birth, Nilakantan crawled under the floor and reinforced the floorboards to make certain the floor would hold the weight.

Another consideration for placement is the water itself. If possible, you should place your tub on linoleum or concrete to prevent the water, which will invariably be tracked out during the birth, from ruining your carpet or wood flooring. An alternative would be to lay a large plastic drop cloth, which can be found at your local hardware or paint store, over the floor to catch the water and protect the wood or carpet.

You also need to make sure you have a clean hose, preferably new, with which to fill and empty the tub. A hose adapter, also available from a hardware store, will allow you to hook your hose directly up to your kitchen sink. You should practice filling and emptying your tub a few times before the actual birth. This will let you know how long it will take to fill, how long the water temperature will hold before you need to add more hot water, and will give you a few trial runs to discover unforeseen problems and deal with them before the birthing event.

Drain your tub by siphoning, or through an existing drain, into a bathtub or shower or, if you live in the country, you can run the water out into the yard. Your tub can then be cleaned and stored for future use, or sent back if it was a rental.

chapter 9
Birth Basics

Every woman's body knows how to give birth, and left to itself, in the majority of cases, would do so without trouble. But not every woman knows or believes this and this self-doubt is often what causes women to be apprehensive and fearful of birth. Making yourself familiar with the nature of birth, and the actual process your body goes through, can help to alleviate these feelings.

The first thing to learn about birth is that it is variable. Just as no two snowflakes are exactly alike, no two births will be either. Don't expect your birth to follow the textbook description as an exact, orderly event. Books about birth were written after taking many births into account and averaging the outcomes. You can apply them to your birth in a general sense, but don't expect your experience to mirror them exactly. Remembering this will help you to feel less anxious when what is happening within your body does not duplicate what you read in a book.

The second thing to learn about birth is that it is a natural and normal process. It is not an illness or a condition that automatically requires medical intervention. Your body is able to give birth just as it is able to pump blood, breathe air, or digest food. These processes are automatic, yet are often affected by other things, like what we do or how we feel. When we are under physical or emotional stress, our heart rate and our rate of respiration go up, while our rate of digestion goes down. Learning to relax and let go of tension at these times does not make these processes work, but it does allow them to work better. Childbirth is like this. There are many things you can do to aid your body in giving birth more easily, even though inherently every woman's body can birth a baby.

The third thing to learn about birth is the actual process. This will allow you to understand what is going on in your body, and this can help you to be more accepting of the physical experience.

Birth is broken into three stages. First, during the dilation stage, your uterus begins the rhythmic tightening and releasing—contractions—that result in the thinning and opening of your cervix, the opening at the base of the uterus that leads to the birth canal. Second, during the pushing stage, your baby is pushed by both the uterine and the abdominal muscles out the cervical opening, between the pelvic bones, down the birth canal, and out. Third, the placenta, which refers to the approximately two and a half pound organ developed during pregnancy for the sole purpose of supporting your baby in the womb, detaches from the sides of the uterus and is pushed out.

Of these three stages, the first, the dilation stage, is the longest and the one women often experience as the most painful part of labor. Once you realize what is happening within your body, this makes sense, as that much squeezing of such a large muscle is bound to produce some pain. Learning to recognize this pain as a natural by-product of your contracting uterus, instead of viewing it as an indication of something wrong, will help you to approach your birth more positively. The dilation stage of labor is also divided into three parts—prelabor, early labor, and active labor.

Pre-labor can last for days, even weeks. This is the preliminary contracting of the uterus that exercises and prepares it for the work ahead. Pre-labor also does the beginning work of early labor, softening and thinning the cervix so that it is ready, once true labor starts, to begin opening. Pre-labor can be exhausting and frustrating. The closer your due date, the more pre-contractions you will have. Sometimes these contractions become so strong and so regular that you think you already are in labor. At that point only a midwife or doctor can tell for sure by checking your cervix. Of course this is not always fail–safe. The day before I had my fourth baby, the midwife said she thought it would be another week. Only your baby knows for sure what day it wants to be born.

When you get a series of these contractions, it is a good idea to rest. Go to your quiet space and lie on your left side. When a contraction comes, try to experience it without judging. Feel the sensation of the tightening and focus on relaxing all of your muscles and on breathing slowly and deeply through it. You will find this very restful as well as being good practice for the birthing. After a while, if it is only pre-labor, your body should slow down and the contractions should stop. If they don't, don't worry about it; just get up and go about your day, doing whatever you need to and rest whenever you need to.

Pre-labor moves gradually into early labor. Sometimes the difference is not easily detected. You may or may not notice the change. When mine switched over to true labor, I noticed that I began having what felt like a cramp in the lower half of my stomach as an accompaniment to the contractions. Before I had my third baby, I had this cramp off and on all day. I didn't know I was in labor because, on checking me that morning, the midwife said that nothing was happening, but that my condition could move into labor at some point. All day long, the cramp came and went. Late that night when I couldn't sleep, the midwife checked me again and found I was definitely in labor and already six centimeters dilated. So, it is not always easy to know when it is true labor and when it is only "practice."

True labor differs from pre-labor in that the contractions you feel are now beginning the job of birthing your baby. Every contraction you get in true labor helps to soften and open you up so that the baby can come through.

In order to understand this process better, it might help to think of your uterus as a large blown-up balloon made up of very strong, flexible muscle fibers. Pear-shaped, it narrows down to a long neck that is your cervix. Tightly closed at the end is the cervical opening that leads to the birth canal.

During each contraction of true labor the muscles at the top of your uterus tighten up, bunching together, causing the muscles along the sides of your uterus to be drawn up, shortening or "thinning" the long neck of the cervix. This process is called "effacing."

Imagining your balloon again, if you were to squeeze the top of the balloon together, it would push the air inside down, making the neck of the balloon shorter. If you continued squeezing, the long neck would eventually disappear and the pressure from the air inside the balloon, along with the shortening sides, would then cause the end to begin opening. This is what your uterus does during the first part of birth. Each contraction squeezes the top of your uterus, making the cervix thinner, or "effacing," and finally begin opening or "dilating." A fully dilated cervix will be ten centimeters, approximately four inches, across, or about the same size around as a Planters twenty-ounce peanut container.

It is usually during the dilation stage that the amniotic sac breaks, although this is not always the case. Sometimes it breaks before labor begins, and sometimes it doesn't break until after the baby's head is born. It is common practice in a medical birth to have the amniotic sac broken by the practitioner sometime during the dilation stage. In a natural birth, they usually let nature take its course unless there is a compelling reason to break the sac, such as labor slowing down, because breaking the sac can stimulate contractions.

In the very early stages of true labor there is still no need to do anything special. Hang out around your house, get things set up, take a walk, rest, watch a movie, do the dishes, do whatever you feel like doing to pass the time. The first part is a lot of waiting without the need to be focused on the birthing.

Active labor begins once you are between four and six centimeters dilated. Once it kicks in, you will know it. The energy of your labor will shift and the contractions will become stronger and more regular. Once my active labor started, I began pacing, walking back and forth, breathing deeply during the contractions, focusing on relaxing and opening. The tub would be filling and I could hear this, and soon all I wanted was to get into the water. I knew instinctively that it would help me to feel better.

When my cervix was dilated to six or seven centimeters, I would get in the water. Getting in any earlier seemed to relax me so much that my labor would slow down. For the next few hours when the contractions grew intense, I labored in the water. Squatting, breathing, focusing on opening, relaxing.

The third part of the dilation phase of labor is called transition. Widely considered the most difficult time of birth, "transition" refers to the relatively short period of time that it takes for your uterus to dilate the last two or three centimeters. Characterized by contractions that are very painful, close together, and longer than they had been, it is during transition that you are most likely to feel that you can't do it. These contractions can feel like you are riding a wave and it's all you can do just to keep your head above the water. Expect to feel overwhelmed at this stage. As your cervix opens up to the full ten centimeters, your body and mind are opening up to allow this new soul to enter the world. I believe that is why the last stage is so intense: it is a surrendering and opening.

During these contractions, it is helpful to breathe very deeply and fully and to make sounds. Opening your mouth and just expelling a sustained "Ahhhh" during the contractions can help to keep you from tightening up your perineum. "Ooomm" is also good, though it takes a little more thought. Whatever sound you make, let it be an opening and expanding sound and one that works with the birthing energy, instead of fighting against it. By the time you have reached transition, your labor is almost over. It is important to try to remember this, as it can help you to get through this intense period.

Once you have made it through transition and your uterus is fully dilated, the energy of the birthing shifts again, marking the beginning of the pushing stage. Now, at the peak of each contraction, you will feel the urge to push. The first evidence of this shift is the tightening of the muscles at the back of the throat as you close off your windpipe and bear down. It is common to make a grunting sound or a tight holding sound followed by a release. Many women feel a very distinctive change in their contractions and in their mental state once this stage begins. Differing from dilation contractions, pushing contractions are longer in duration and usually farther apart. Many women find them less painful and, after the helpless feeling that often accompanies transition, they often welcome this more active phase where they can actively participate in the birth of their baby.

During the pushing stage, both the uterus and the mother work hard in conjunction to push the baby through the cervix into the birth canal, down between the pelvic bones and to the opening of the vagina where the baby's head first appears or "crowns." The length of time it takes for the baby's head to crown varies but is typically shorter if you are having a waterbirth and typically longer if you had an epidural. The average pushing stage for a waterbirth is 25 minutes; the average for a woman who has had an epidural is 60 to 90 minutes. It is just as the head crowns that an episiotomy, a cut in the wall of the perineum to prevent tearing, is usually given. In a waterbirth, as the warm water has helped to soften the perineum tissue making it more pliable and able to stretch, episiotomies are rarely needed.

In most cases, a baby's head is presenting and comes out first. As you push the baby out, you will feel a lot of pressure as the head moves down and a burning, searing pain as your perineum stretches. Stay focused and breathe. At this point it is almost over and the baby will be here at last. Birthing the baby's head is the most intense part as the rest of the baby is smaller and more pliable. Once the head comes out, if you are having a waterbirth, you can reach down and feel it, welcoming your baby. I always loved this part, being able to have the first contact with my baby even before it was fully born.

Once the head is born, the baby turns slightly to allow each shoulder to come out, one after the other. While this happens, do not push too hard, instead breathe fast and light and allow the baby's shoulders to come out one at a time. This will reduce the risk of the perineum tearing, the risk of which is already considerably reduced by your being in the water. If you are having a conventional hospital birth, the doctors will probably have already given you an episiotomy.

Once the shoulders have been born, the rest of the baby will slide out easily.

If you are birthing in water, once born, the baby must be brought up out of the water either by yourself or the attendant. There are some people who like to let the baby stay under water for a while after the birth, but I never had the patience for that. After nine months of waiting, I wanted to see and hold my baby.

If you are birthing in the hospital and do not want your baby to be taken from you immediately after birth, be sure to let them know beforehand that that is what you want. In most cases they will allow you to keep the baby with you on your bare skin for the first moments after birth. They will at some point want to take the baby away to clean and weigh it, but try to preserve as much time with your infant after the birth as you can. There is no need to weigh the baby immediately; it will weigh the same an hour after birth as it does at birth. And the baby doesn't care if it is clean; all it wants is the closeness and security of its mother.

If you are waterbirthing, your baby is already washed clean of blood and is weightless, and you can remain in the tub for as long as you like.

A short while after your baby is born, you will feel the urge to push again. This signals that you are ready to deliver the placenta, which may be birthed directly into the water, or into a bowl while you remain standing in the water, or you may get out of the tub altogether to deliver the placenta. During the births of my first four children, I got out of the tub to deliver the placenta. After my fifth baby was born, I delivered the placenta into a bowl while I remained standing in the tub. This was a nice change as I was then able to sit back down in the water and play with my baby.

Sometime during your delivery, the umbilical cord will be cut. Attached to the placenta at one end and the baby at the other, the umbilical cord acted to bring nourishment to, and to remove wastes from, the baby while *in utero.* In a medical birth, the cord is cut almost immediately after the baby is born. In a natural birth, it is generally not cut until after the cord has stopped pulsing, signaling that the nutrient rich maternal blood is no longer flowing to the baby.

This completes the birth process. After this, you will be cleaned up and settled wherever you wish in order to rest and to begin the lifelong process of motherhood.

The final thing to learn about birth is that there are many things you can do to make your experience of birth less painful and more rewarding. Some of them are learned, such as the breathing and relaxation techniques taught in prenatal yoga and other childbirth education classes. Others are instinctual, which require your recognizing and respecting them, such as honoring the urge to walk or squat or sway during contractions. Other aids are topical, such as warm pools of water, hot showers, massage, and counter pressure to your lower back, which help to directly ease the pain and remind you to relax. Others, still, are environmental like having an appropriate place to give birth where you feel safe and secure, with family and close friends around you for support.

Each of these can contribute to easing the pain you may feel during your labor, offering you a solid support system should you choose to give birth naturally. This moves us into the next stage of planning for your birth: The Preparation.

Part II

The Preparation

chapter 10

Yoga for Pregnancy

During your birth your resources are going to be tapped out, much as if you were running a long marathon. Everything you know and everything you are will be utilized to see you through this challenging experience. However you decide to meet this challenge, at home or in the hospital, with pain reduction from drugs or from water labor and delivery, you are going to benefit from having learned a few techniques to see you through. In the same way you would train for a marathon, you can train for your birth.

Prenatal yoga, by teaching you to be aware of your body, and how to breathe effectively, and how to consciously relax, is one way for you to train for your birth. The poses themselves, by gently strengthening and stretching the muscles most commonly used during birth (those of the abdomen and pelvic region), prepare your body for the stress of the birth. The relaxation effect produced is used both during the pregnancy to keep exhaustion at bay and during the birth for rejuvenation. The breathing techniques show you how to use your breath as a focal point during labor to produce a calming effect, or as a powerful energizer to keep your strength up.

Mentally, the practice of the poses and techniques taught in yoga will create in you a feeling of deep peace. Almost from the very first session, as you move slowly through each pose, you will feel a tranquility settle over you. By the end of the session during the deep relaxation exercise, as your thoughts subside and your worries fade, you will slip easily into a totally relaxed state, reaching a level of relaxation that you may have not felt in years.

Here, in this deep-relaxed state, having been gently exercised, your body will begin repairing anything amiss within your system. If you practice these poses regularly, your body will continue to heal, eventually becoming completely renewed. It is this healing benefit that has made the practice of yoga a central part of the work of both Dr. Dean Ornish and his program for preventing and reversing heart disease, and Dr. Deepak Chopra who, through his books and centers, has been successfully treating many illnesses ranging from stress-related ulcers to cancer.

During the delicate condition of pregnancy the regular practice of yoga will help keep your health up by supporting the systems of your body that are additionally taxed from this stressful, though natural, condition. As you continue to practice, you will notice that you feel more balanced, more relaxed, not only during the yoga session, but also at other times throughout the day. You will begin to feel an overall sense of calm, a renewed ability to handle the stresses of your life and to meet challenges more readily. Your body will feel strong and healthy, your mind serene.

The following series of yoga poses and stretches are the ones I did during my pregnancies and again, with a few modifications, after the babies were born. Included with the descriptions of these exercises are details of their benefits.

If you have not practiced yoga before, you need to wait until after you have entered your fourth month before you begin the class. Waiting until this time means the greatest risk of miscarriage has passed, and it will allow you to have recovered from most of the nausea and exhaustion that typically accompany the first three months. There are some exceptions to this rule. The breathing and relaxation techniques may be started at any time. They do not pose any risk to you or the baby and are useful in helping you to feel less tired. Other poses that may be started immediately are noted in the instruction portion of each exercise.

If you have been practicing yoga regularly for at least six months prior to becoming pregnant, you can continue to practice under the guidance of a qualified yoga teacher.

If you have any health condition related to or independent of the pregnancy that prohibits your exercising, you should show this prenatal class, described in the next chapter, to your practitioner and get approval prior to beginning the class.

chapter 11

How To Begin

Yoga should be done regularly, at least two to three times a week, and is ideally done daily, to reap the most benefit. If you find yourself short of time, or are too tired to do a complete class, at least do the relaxation exercise, as this is the single most important technique you can practice to help you have a more comfortable pregnancy, a more positive birth experience, and an easier recovery period once the baby is born.

Contrary to traditional yoga practices which recommend you abstain from food or drink before you practice, for prenatal yoga it is recommended that you eat a small snack within thirty to forty-five minutes of beginning. This will keep you from feeling dizzy or nauseous from exercising on an empty stomach while pregnant. If at any time you do feel dizzy or nauseous, stop the class and lie down on your left side, to allow for the optimal blood flow to the baby, and take a few slow, deep breaths to relax. Remember that your body will not be as reliable as usual during your pregnancy. One day you may sail through the entire class feeling energetic and vibrant, while the next day even the slightest movement will make you feel exhausted. Always listen to your body and do what it tells you. Not only will this prevent you from overdoing it while you are pregnant, but it will also develop this self-awareness into a habit which will come in useful during your birthing.

Your practice surface should be soft, preferably carpeted. A mat or blanket may be laid over a bare floor if you do not have carpeting, but care must be taken to make sure you do not slip during the standing poses and the ones done by the wall. For the class, you will need three or four pillows that will be used at various times. Set them beside your practice area at the beginning of the class so you will have them at hand when you need them.

Once you are ready to start, begin slowly. As you practice regularly you will be able to increase the duration of the poses and the number of times each pose repeats. But in the beginning err on the side of caution and always stop at about half the maximum that you feel you can do. Yoga is not like other exercises in that you prove their worth by how well you can do them. The benefit of yoga comes from the manner in which each pose is done, as well as from the pose itself. This is why the simplest beginner can reap much the same benefit as the advanced practitioner.

During the class always remain aware of your body. Never strain or over–stretch during the class. Pay close attention to how each movement feels. As you move through the poses notice which parts of your body feel strong and which feel weak, which are tight and which are flexible. Becoming aware of how your body feels during each pose allows you to begin modifying your body, making the weak parts stronger, and the tight parts more flexible, and allowing you to achieve an overall sense of balance throughout your physique.

This awareness of your body is a fringe benefit of practicing yoga. By being aware during pregnancy you recognize the many changes that are taking place, and are able to adapt to them more readily. Being aware of your body also means being aware of your baby, giving you the daily opportunity to consciously focus on your baby growing inside you.

chapter 12

Prenatal Yoga Class

Begin by taking a comfortable seated position. As your pregnancy progresses, you may find that sitting in a chair is no longer comfortable as your legs can swell from hanging over the sides of your chair. Learning a few comfortable positions for sitting on the floor will give you an alternative to chair sitting.

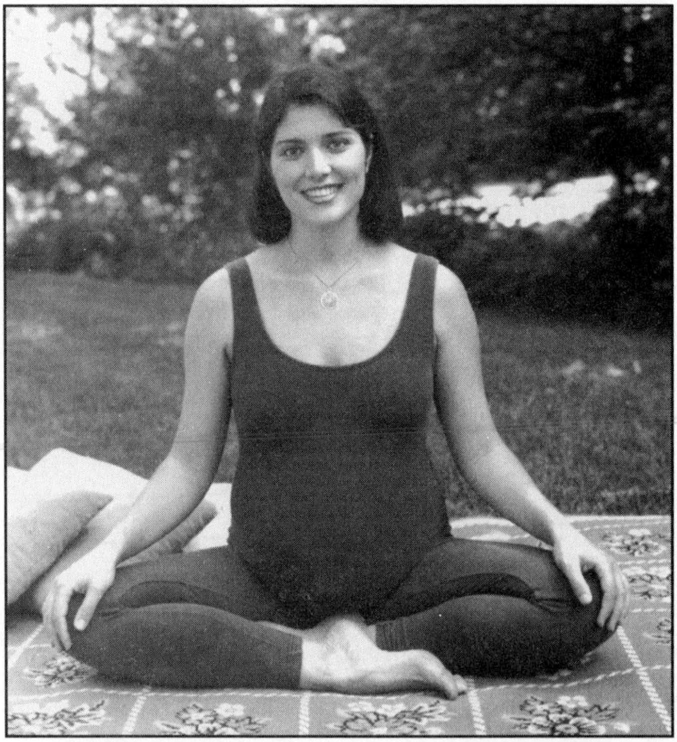

On the floor, sit with your legs crossed. If this is not comfortable, place a pillow under your buttocks to elevate your hips. A pillow placed here can help you to sit up straighter and it removes some of the strain from your hip joints. You may also place a pillow under each leg, to support your knees.

Adjust your position until you feel the most comfortable. Close your eyes and sit up straight, feeling as if you are lifting

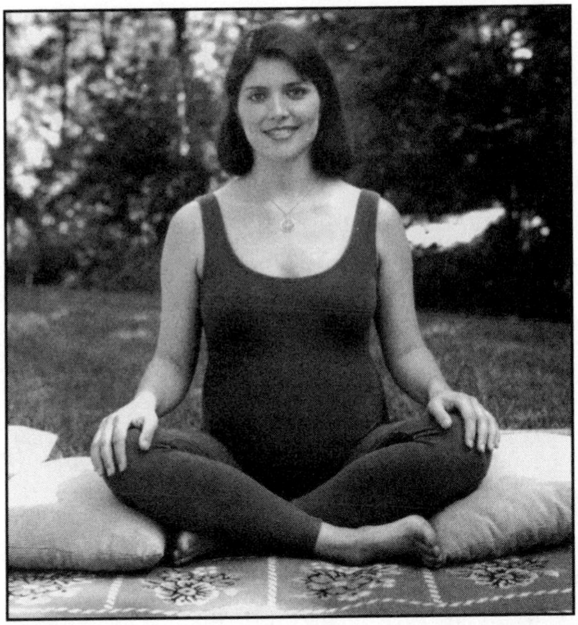

from the center of your head all the way along your spine toward the ceiling. Inhale slowly and deeply and exhale in the same relaxed manner. Do this three times, feeling as though you are letting go, releasing all of your tension with each exhalation and bringing focus and awareness in with each inhalation.

Neck stretches: Still seated, inhale; as you exhale, slowly drop your chin to your chest. Hold this position for a moment, breathing normally. Then, on an inhalation, raise your head back to center. On your next exhalation, bend your head to the right, right ear toward right shoulder, hold, inhale, and raise to center. Exhale, left ear toward left shoulder, inhale, and raise to center. Repeat this sequence two more times, focusing on gently stretching and feeling the release of tension in this area; stop when you raise your head to the center again.

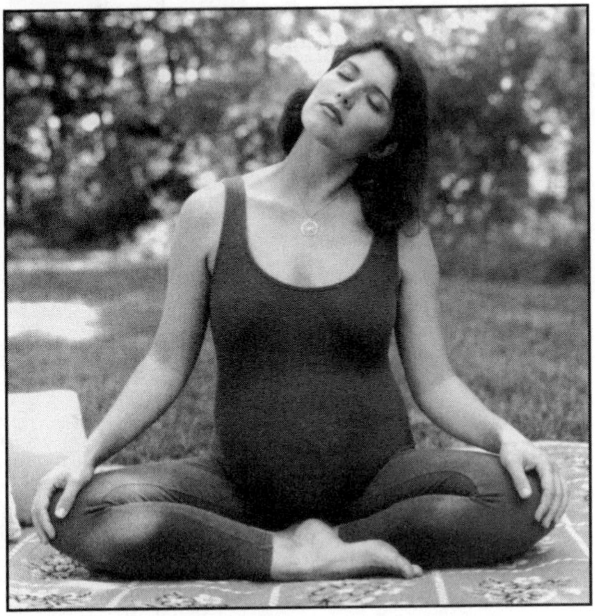

Neck rolls: Inhale, exhale, bring your chin to your chest to center, hold; as you inhale this time, roll your head to the side until your right ear is over your right shoulder; exhale, roll back to center; inhale, roll to the left. Finish by raising your head to center. Repeat three times each way.

Generally, if you find that you carry a lot of tension in

your neck, build up to doing eight to ten repetitions for this exercise and repeat throughout out the day. Don't push it, as you could give yourself a headache or a sore neck.

BENEFITS: Neck stretches and rolls are good for releasing tension in the back of your neck, something you are likely to experience a lot as your girth increases. The muscles in the back of your neck attach to the muscles that expand around your abdomen, so as your stomach gets bigger, those muscles pull on your neck muscles and cause them to get tighter. Regularly stretching your neck muscles can prevent the accompanying tension and strain that can result.

Shoulder rolls: Raise your hands so your fingertips rest lightly on your shoulders. Have your elbows lead the movement, bringing them forward, up, back, and down, making a complete circle. Focus on moving slowly and fully through the movement. Do three repetitions, then reverse the process, rolling forward.

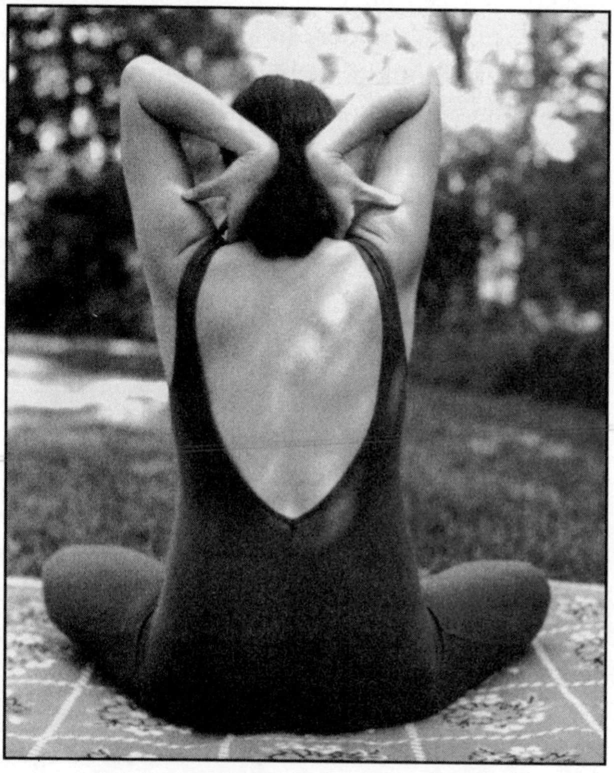

BENEFITS: This exercise relaxes and strengthens the muscles of the shoulders and upper back. They also help to maintain good posture. Your arms will be used for everything once the baby is born and you are likely to develop what I call "nurser's syndrome." This refers to the tightness in your arms, neck, and shoulders, and the accompanying aching and cramping that come from carrying the baby all the time, bending over the baby all the time, and looking at the baby all the time while the baby is lying in your arms and breast- or bottle-feeding. The symptoms of "nurser's syndrome" are headaches, neck pain, upper back and shoulder pain, rounded or hunched back, aching arms, and irritability. Palliating these are neck and shoulder rolls that strengthen, stretch, and tone the muscles in the affected region.

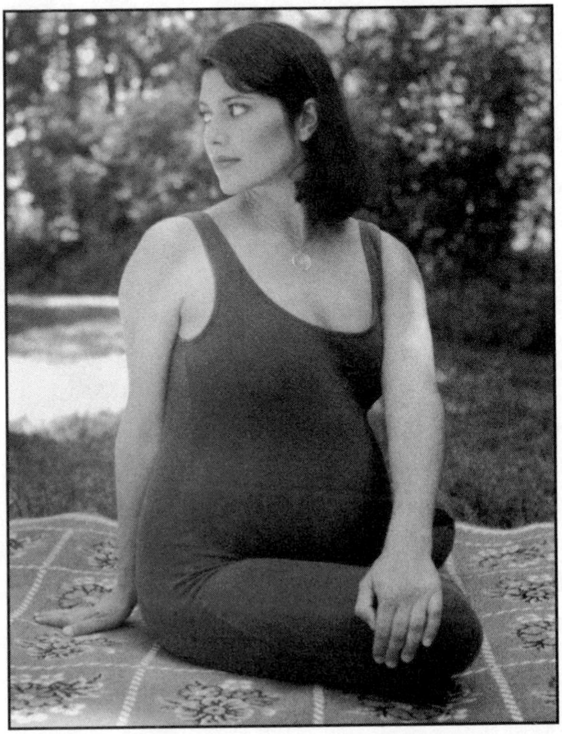

Half-Spinal Twist: Remain in your cross-legged position. Inhale; then as you exhale, bring your left hand to your right knee, turn your upper body to the right and look over your right shoulder. Place your right hand or fingertips on the floor behind you at the base of your spine, completing the twist. While in the pose, breathe deeply and really relax into it, twisting a little further on your exhalation. Always be careful not to push yourself too far. Hold this position for 20 to 25 seconds, then inhale, and as you exhale, turn back to center. Twist to the left by inhaling; on your exhalation, turn your body to the left, grasping your left knee with your right hand. Look over your left shoulder as your left hand comes to rest at the base of your spine behind you. Hold for 20 to 25 seconds. Inhale, exhale, and return to center.

BENEFITS: This stretch increases the mobility of the spine and gives a gentle massage to the liver, kidneys, and adrenals, improving their ability to function properly. It also helps to correct the posture and to relieve tension carried between the shoulder blades.

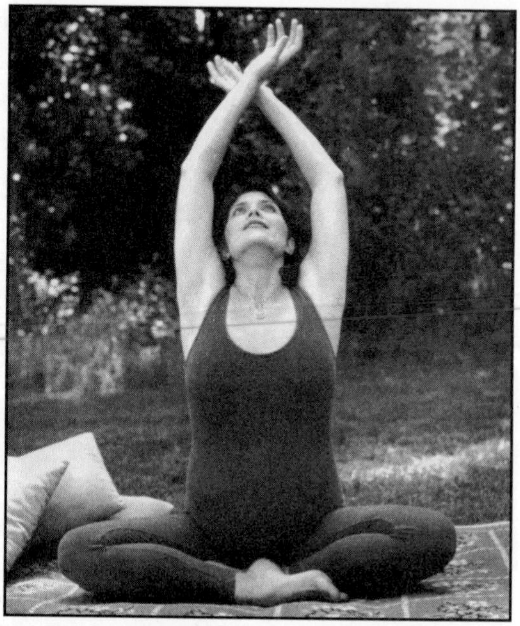

Cleansing Breath: Inhale as deeply as you can. On your exhalation, open your mouth and let the air rush out. As you do this, incorporate a sound: for instance, "Ahhhh." Inhale, and as you exhale say, "Ahhhh." Any open sound may be used, such as "Ohhhh" or "Uuuuu." Let the sound be open and loose, coming through a relaxed mouth and jaw. You may raise your arms on the inhalation, letting them drop on the exhalation as a variation. Repeat this breath one to three times.

BENEFITS: The cleansing breath allows you to release any tension you may have built up during the pose, and is also deeply relaxing. Taking such a deep breath causes your collarbones to rise. This releases a chemical into your brain telling your body to relax. Doing this breath any time you feel tension or stress will make you feel more relaxed. We will be doing a number of cleansing breaths throughout the class, but it can also be done anytime in your day that you feel stress or tension.

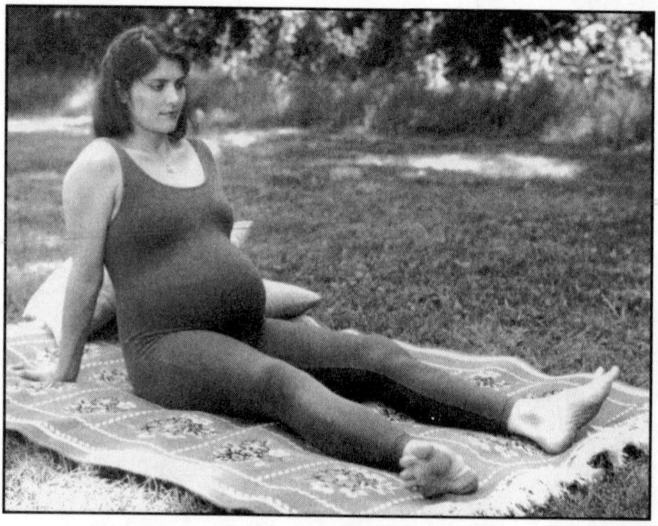

Stretch and Roll: Whenever your legs become tight or uncomfortable in your seated position, you may stretch them out in front of you and roll them from side to side.

BENEFITS: This will release any built-up tension in your hips and legs.

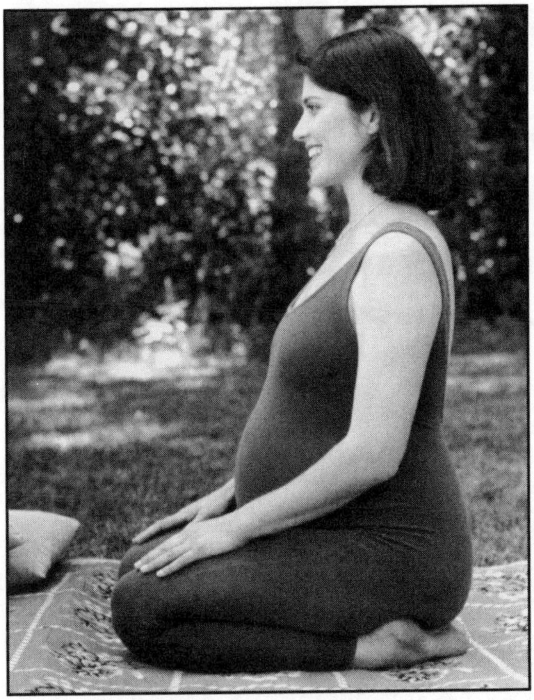

Diamond Pose: Come up onto your knees into a kneeling position. Make sure your knees and feet are close together. Allowing your toes to remain together, let your heals fall apart. Sit back on your heels. As a variation, place a pillow on your feet and under your buttocks, and sit back on the pillow. Sit in this position for 45 to 60 seconds.

BENEFITS: The diamond pose lifts and opens the diaphragm, giving you more "room" as your abdomen expands, making it a good position to sit in frequently during the first three months when nausea and indigestion ("morning sickness") can cause so much discomfort. It also helps the blood from the legs to return to the heart, and helps to prevent edema (water retention) in the legs.

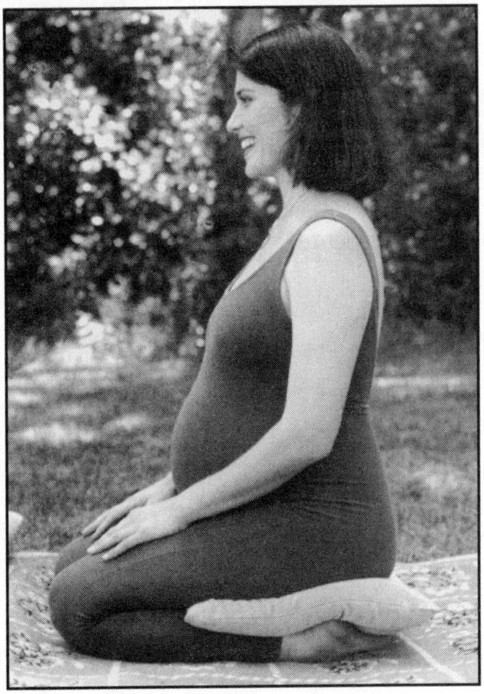

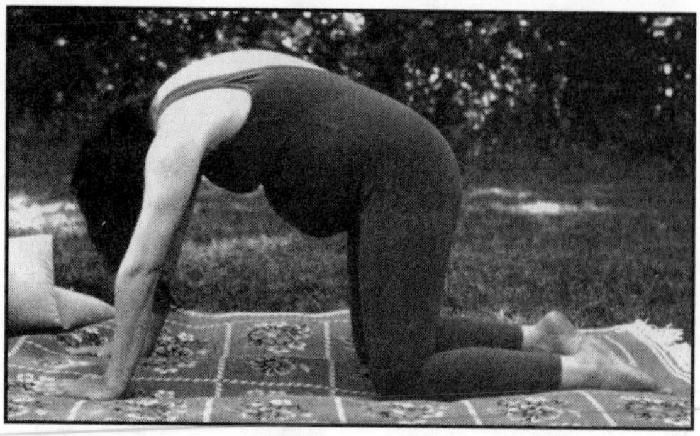

Cat/Cow: Sit forward on all fours in the "table" position. See that your back is straight and that your knees and hands are directly under your hips and shoulders and about shoulder width apart. Inhale; as you exhale, slowly tuck your pelvis under, arching your back and bringing your chin down to your chest. Exhale fully.

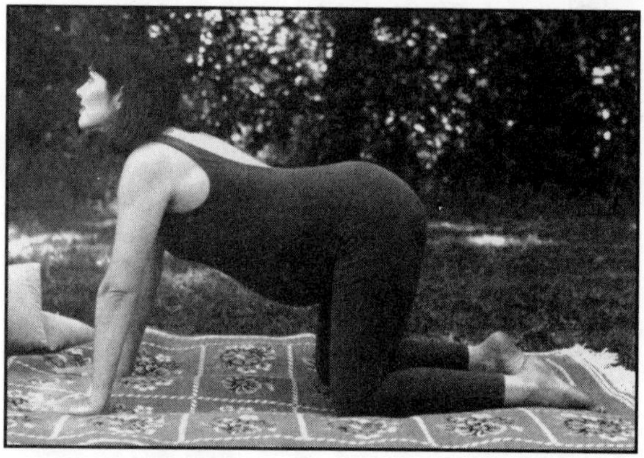

Now, inhale, opening back up the other way; tilt your pelvis up and your belly towards the floor as your head raises up to look toward the ceiling. Repeat eight to ten times each way, gradually increasing this number as you feel comfortable. Come out of the pose by sitting back onto your heels in the diamond position.

CAUTION: While performing the cat/cow, it is very important that you do not dip your belly down too far, as this could cause you to pull the ligaments on either side of your lower abdomen. As opposed to trying to dip deep, think instead of elongating your spine in both directions and making a gentle curve with your back.

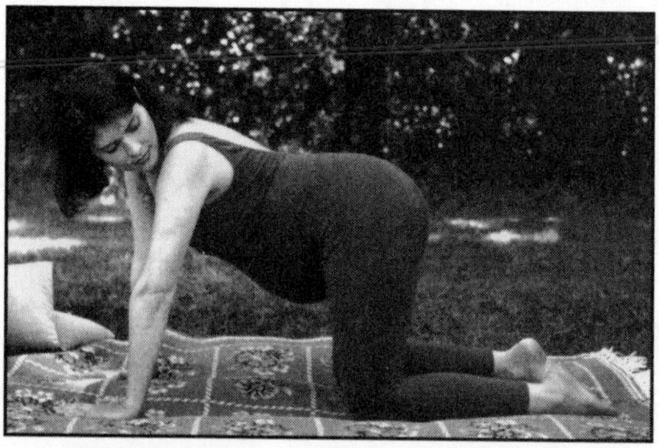

Variation: Coming back into the table position, elongate your spine; inhale, and as you exhale, bring your right shoulder and your right hip towards each other; look over your right shoulder back to your hip, making a C curve with your body. Inhale and come back to center. Exhale and bend to the left. As you do this make sure to keep your back flat and your spine elongated. Repeat eight to ten times.

BENEFITS: Both the traditional cat/cow and its variation relieve tension in your lower back and in the rest of your spine by keeping them flexible and relaxed. This position takes the pressure of the growing baby off the pelvic floor, easing tension and giving those muscles a well-needed break. It strengthens the sides of the waist and the muscles of the lower back and abdomen.

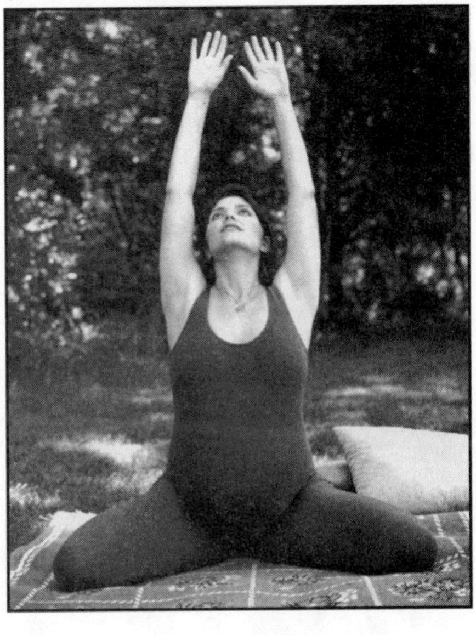

Folded Pose: Sitting back onto your heels again as in the diamond pose, inhale, raise your arms above your head, and stretch.

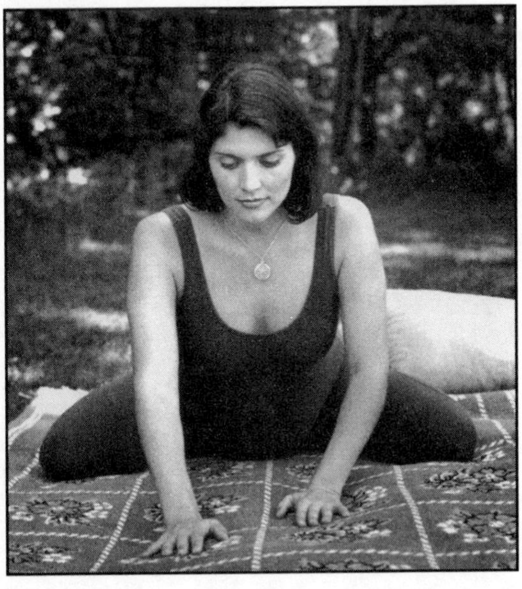

Open your knees wide and as you exhale, bring your hands to the floor in front of you and "walk" yourself down to the floor, until your upper body rests between your open legs.

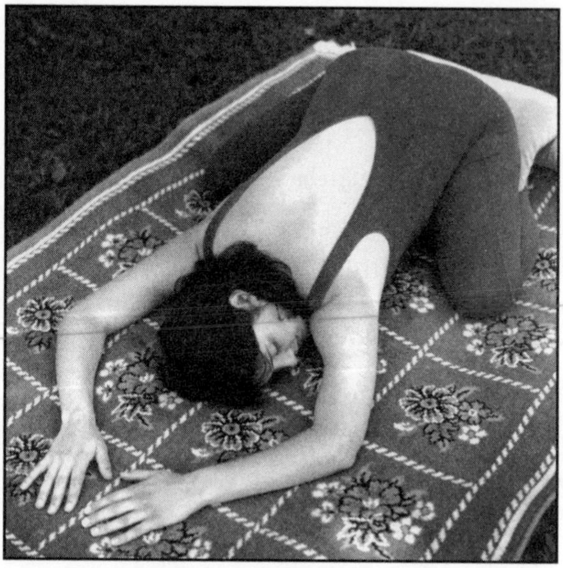

Go down as far as is comfortable, and relax. You may place a pillow under your buttocks, and/or under your chest to make this position more comfortable. Stay in this position for 45 seconds to a minute, or longer, if it is comfortable for you. To come out of this pose, slowly "walk" yourself to the upright position, allowing your head to come up last.

BENEFITS: This pose relieves the pressure of the growing baby on the pelvic floor. It provides relaxation for the lower spine, and it gives a gentle stretch to the inner thighs. It is one of my favorite positions to rest in during labor, both during and in between contractions.

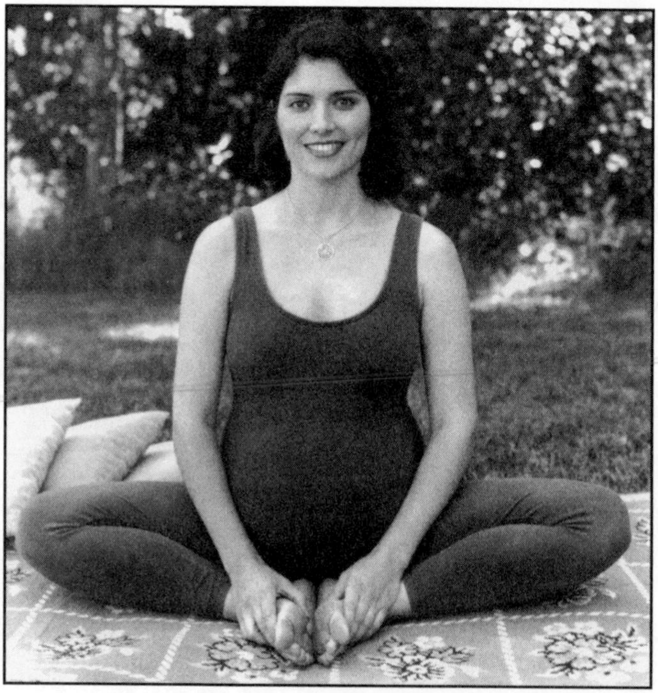

Butterfly: Sit up straight in your cross–legged position, then bring the soles of your feet together in front of you, close in to your body. Taking hold of the toes, relax the knees out. You may place pillows under each knee if this position is uncomfortable for your hips. Inhale, sit up straighter, and gently press your knees towards the floor.

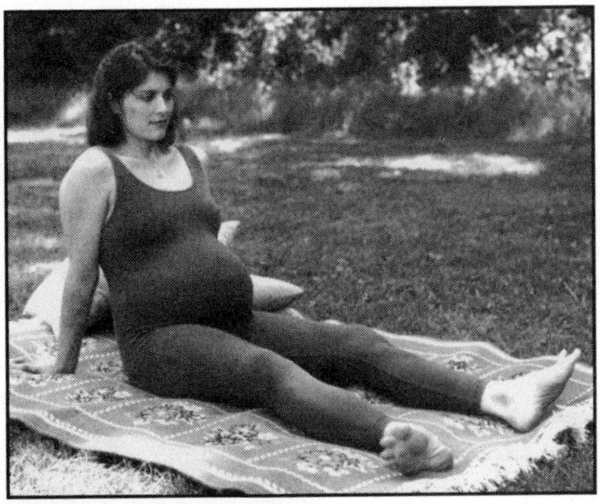

Hold for a minute, then stretch your legs out in front of you and roll them from side to side.

BENEFITS: The butterfly stretches and tones the perineum and the inner thighs. It keeps the hip joints loose and open and is a good pose to practice in preparation for the more demanding upcoming squat.

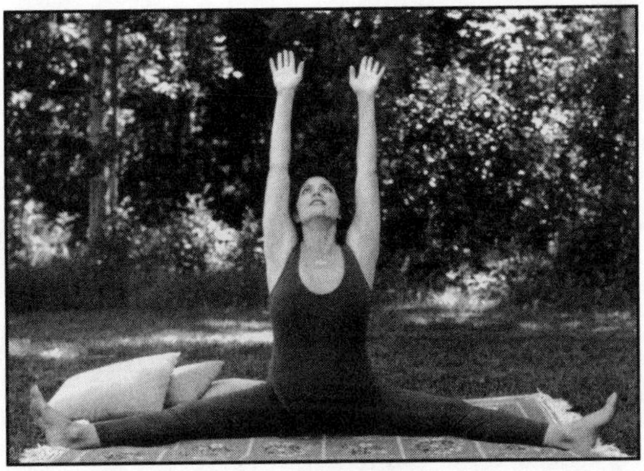

Side Stretch in "V" Position: Coming out of the butterfly, stretch your legs out one at a time until you are in the sitting "V" position. Open your legs as wide as you can without strain. Inhale, stretch your arms above your head, and lift up.

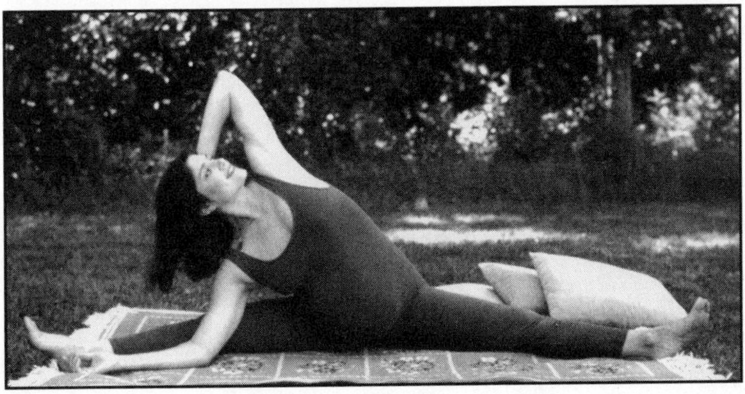

Exhale, bend slowly to the right, bringing your right arm down; then place your right palm on the floor in front of your leg for support. Slide your right hand down your right leg as far as is comfortable. Stretch your left arm up and out over your right leg, feeling the stretch all the way up the side of your body and in your inner thigh.

Hold for 30 seconds, breathe normally, and relax into the stretch. Inhale, lift to center, exhale and bend slowly to the left over the left leg. Rest the left palm on the floor for balance while stretching the right arm up and out over your left leg. Relax into the pose. Breathe deeply and relax into this position, getting used to the feel and the idea of opening.

BENEFITS: This exercise stretches the muscles of the inner thighs and opens the perineum. Getting used to keeping this area relaxed and open will help you during birth when the tendency is to tighten up.

Forward Stretch in "V" Position: Remaining in the "V" position, inhale, stretch your arms above your head, then lift up. Exhale and bring your hands to the floor; slowly begin "walking" your hands forward, coming down into the stretch. Go only so far as is comfortable, then let your chin drop towards your chest to relax. Breathe deeply, feeling the stretch. Hold for 30 seconds, then, "walking" your hands back to center, come up. Take three deep "cleansing breaths" and stretch your legs out, and shake and roll them from side to side, releasing any built-up tension.

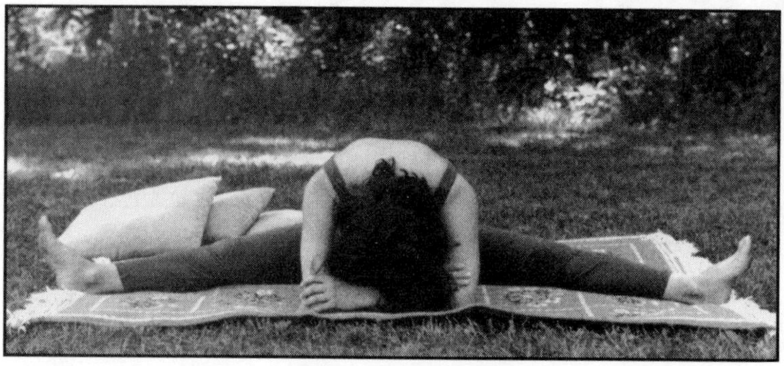

CAUTION: Be careful not to over-stretch in this position. The tendons in your hip joints and pelvis are loose due to hormones being released in your body in preparation for the birth; the looseness makes it easy to stretch beyond your normal capacity. Err on the side of caution and stretch a little less than your ability.

BENEFITS: This exercise stretches the muscles of the inner thighs and opens the perineum.

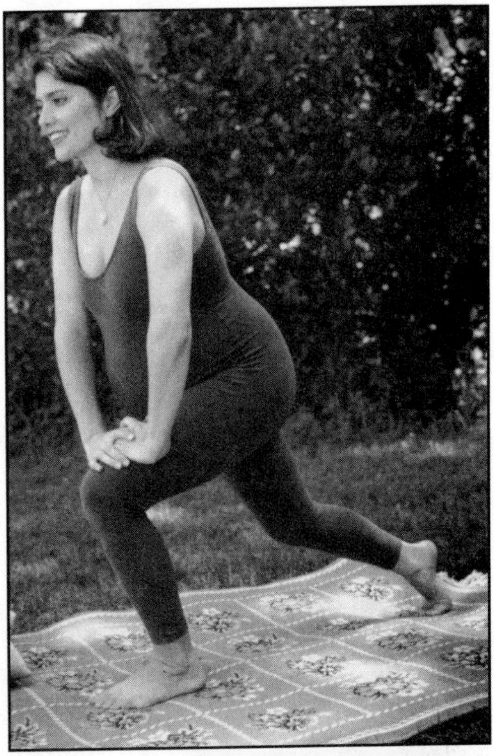

How to get off the floor: This may seem strange, but actually it is very useful as the seated yoga poses are often so comfortable during pregnancy. You may find yourself sitting on the floor much more frequently than normal and having to get up off the floor more often than you would expect. To get up off the floor, come into a kneeling position; bring your left leg forward, placing the sole of your foot on the floor. Curl the toes of your right foot under for support. Place both hands on your right thigh for balance, and push up until you are in a standing position.

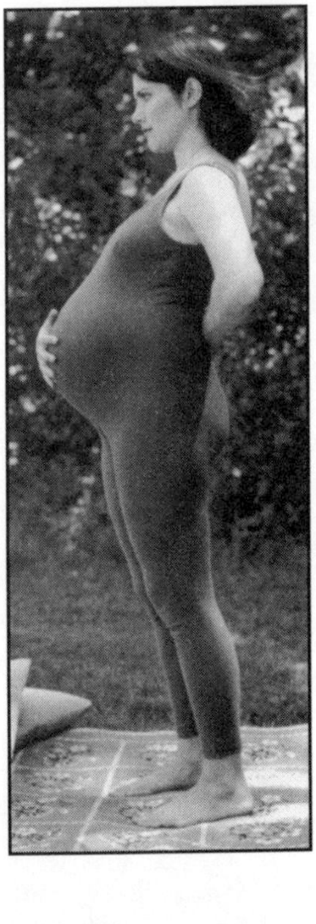

Posture Correction: During pregnancy there is a tendency for your posture to deteriorate. As your baby gets bigger, it pulls your belly forward, placing strain on your lower back, and pulls your shoulders down, causing neck and upper back pain. To correct this, stand with your feet a little wider apart than hip distance; see that they are facing forward and are firmly and evenly planted on the ground. Soften your knees, tuck your pelvis under, pull your belly slightly in, inhale, roll your

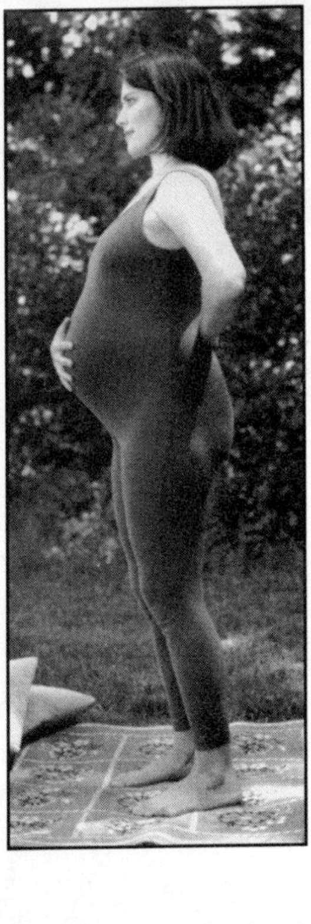

shoulders up and back and down and then stretch up, lifting the center of your head toward the ceiling. Now, stand there a moment to see how this feels. It may feel a little unnatural at first, but the more you practice becoming aware of how you are standing, the easier it will be to remember to maintain good posture.

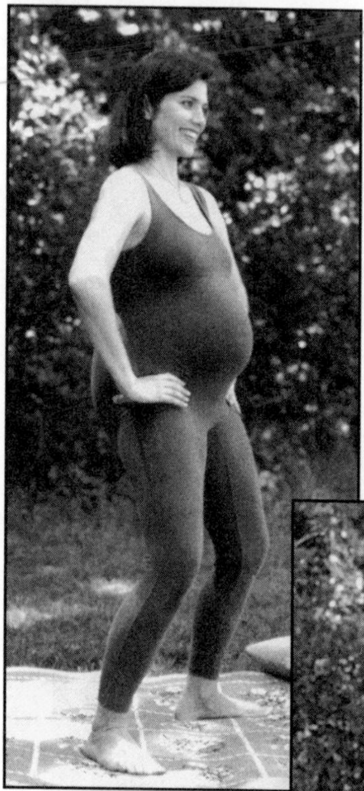

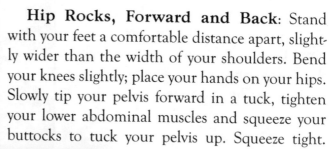

Hip Rocks, Forward and Back: Stand with your feet a comfortable distance apart, slightly wider than the width of your shoulders. Bend your knees slightly; place your hands on your hips. Slowly tip your pelvis forward in a tuck, tighten your lower abdominal muscles and squeeze your buttocks to tuck your pelvis up. Squeeze tight. Then, slowly release and rock back the other way. Sticking your buttocks way back, feel the muscles in your lower back tighten and feel the muscles across the front of your belly stretch and relax. Tipping forward again, feel the relaxation in your lower back as your front tightens again. Repeat this process, front and back, eight to ten times, as is comfortable for you.

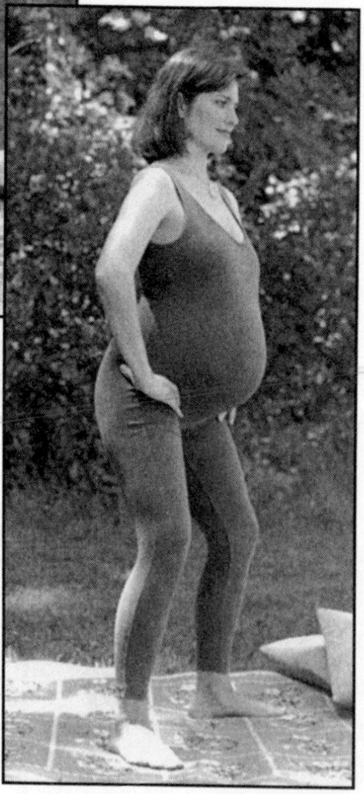

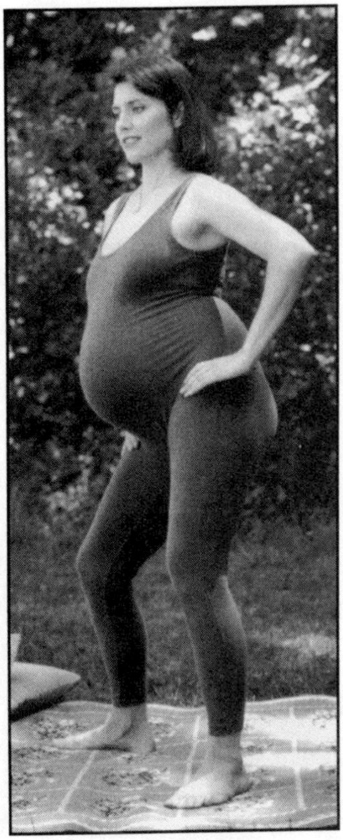

Hip Circles: From the same standing position as you held for the hip rocks, tip your hips to the right, then roll around to the back, roll to the left, and then to the front. Continue rolling, focusing on doing the complete motion for each circle, as if you were doing a hula-hoop. Don't be afraid to move. Do eight to ten repetitions to the right and to the left.

BENEFITS: Hip circles and hip rocks are invaluable in pregnancy. If a pregnant woman does nothing but these exercises, she will greatly relieve her discomfort and increase her ease in giving birth. These exercises tone all the abdominal muscles you will use to carry and birth your baby. In some cultures, these exercises are thought to not only ease birth, but to increase youth and fertility. From my experience, I have found another benefit. By focusing on the part of my body where the greatest changes are taking place, they allow me to notice these changes and relate to them positively. It feels so good to roll through hip circles with such a large belly, to rock back and forth as if I were rocking my baby. After the baby is born, these same exercises will help to strengthen and tighten the muscles of the abdomen and lower back.

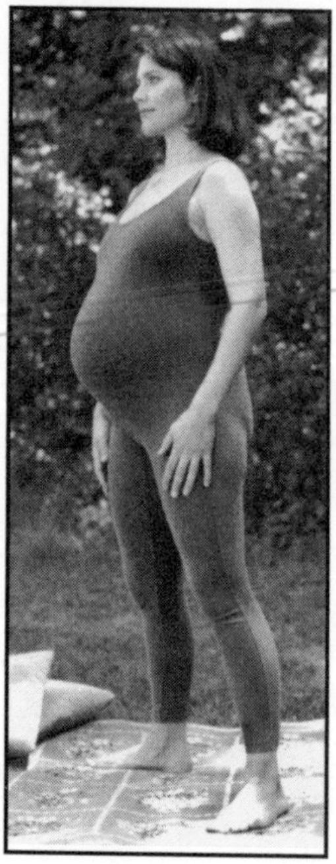

Squat: Assume the same beginning position as you took for the hip rocks and hip circles, then inhale, and, as you exhale, slide your hands down your legs, bending at the knees until you are all the way down into a squat. Push your legs apart slightly to accommodate your belly.

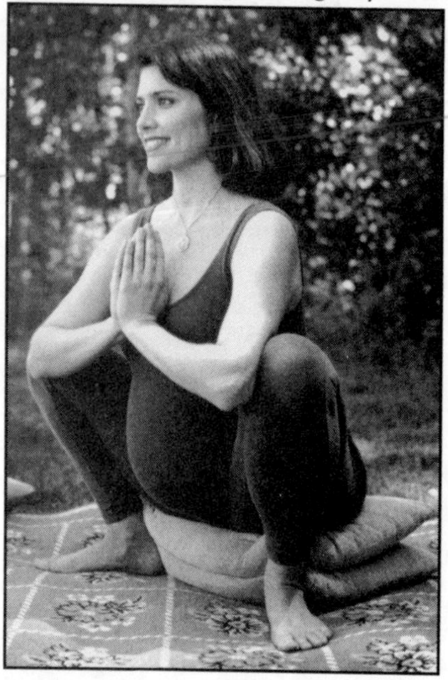

Stay in this position for 45 to 60 seconds.

To come out of the squat, bring your hands to the floor in front of you, drop your head and slowly raise your buttocks to the ceiling. Then roll up slowly to a standing position. Stay there for a moment, regaining your balance, then do three cleansing breaths.

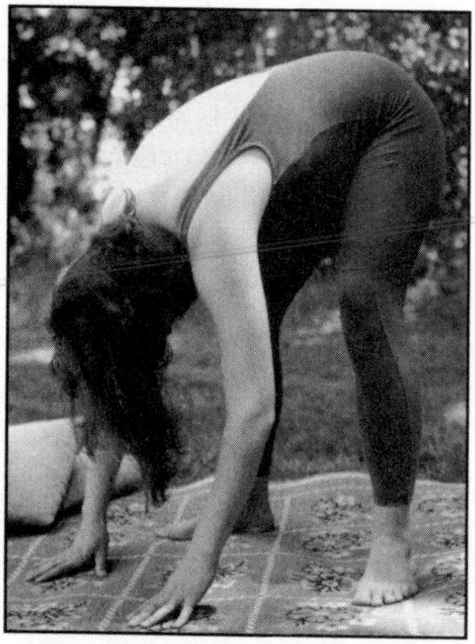

Modified Squat: If you find that doing a full squat isn't comfortable for you, place pillows under your buttocks to give you extra support.

CAUTION: Do not do a full squat if you have hemorrhoids as the pressure on your rectum can push the hemorrhoids out. Instead, do a modified squat against the wall with pillows under your buttocks. This will give you the opening, stretching benefits of the squat without putting undue pressure on your rectum.

BENEFITS: Squatting has many benefits both for your pregnancy and in terms of birth. Because of this, you should squat often, not just during this class. If at first you aren't able to go all the way down, practice (and keep practicing) until it becomes comfortable for you. Practicing in a large bath or a swimming pool is sometimes easier if you have access to these. You can also squat while you work in the garden; while you dress your toddler; while you hang out with a friend.

Squatting stretches and tones the muscles of the upper thighs and the perineum, making them strong and supple. It allows the muscles of the lower back to relax by relieving the pressure and weight of the growing baby on your lower spine and pelvic region. It is the best position to be in during the pushing stage of your birth as squatting actually shortens the birth canal, and being in the upright position allows for the natural pull of gravity to help you to birth your baby more easily. Squatting during labor eases back pain during the contractions, and it can help to stimulate contractions by allowing your baby's head to press more fully onto the cervix.

In a waterbirth, squatting is very comfortable. I gave birth to four of my children in the squatting position. The fifth baby had a shoulder briefly stuck. I gave birth to her on all fours, which allowed her shoulder to slide out easily.

Kegels: Kegels are another exercise which can be done at any time and whose benefits cannot be stressed enough. Kegels, so named for the doctor who first developed them, are practiced by squeezing the muscles of the perineum and rectum very tightly, then holding for three to five seconds, and releasing. To make sure you are doing this exercise correctly, you can try it first while you pee. While peeing, tighten the muscles you would use to stop the flow of your urine. If you can stop the flow completely, your muscles are in good shape. If you can slow it down, but not stop it completely, your muscles are a little weak and need strengthening. If you aren't able to slow the flow at all, your muscles need a lot of work.

Begin by doing twenty to twenty-five kegels during this class, and then another twenty to twenty-five every time you pee. The recommendation is that you build up in this manner until you are doing two to three hundred kegels a day. That may seem like a lot, but if you consider doing twenty kegels every time you pee, which is about ten times a day for a pregnant woman, you will have done two hundred kegels. The other thing about kegels that makes doing so many of them realistic is that, as they are done completely internally, you can do them any time, anywhere, and no one will know you are doing them.

BENEFITS: Kegels strengthen all the muscles of the pelvic floor, keeping them strong and healthy during pregnancy and toning them up for the birth. Muscles that are in good shape stretch easier, tear less, and recover more quickly after the baby is born. Doing this exercise will also familiarize you with how your pelvic muscles feel when they are tight and how they feel when they are relaxed, and this will help you determine, while giving birth, if you are unconsciously tightening up. They also teach you to relax your pelvic floor on demand, a skill that will allow your cervix to open up more easily during your birth.

Moon Sequence: This is a sequence of poses that moves one way, working one side of the body, and then moves back the other way, working the other side. They are to be done in succession, flowing one into the next, without breaking the movement. Begin by standing with your feet apart, facing forward.

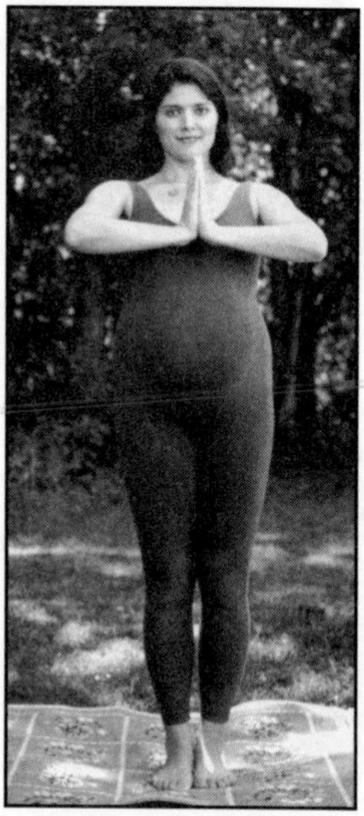

Position one: hands in prayer mode at the chest.

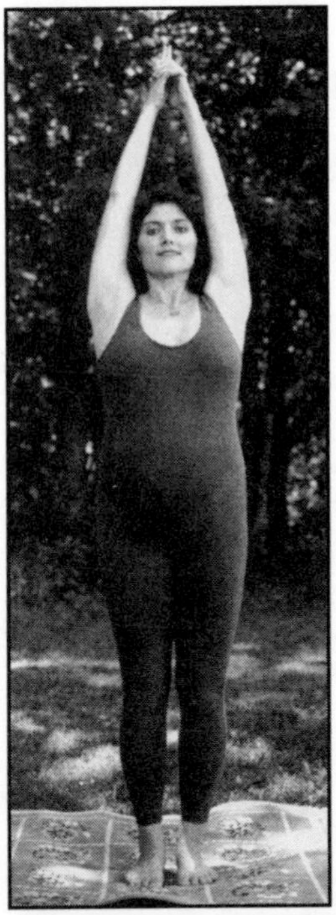

Position two: raise your arms overhead with the palms together in steeple position.

Position three: bend to the right.

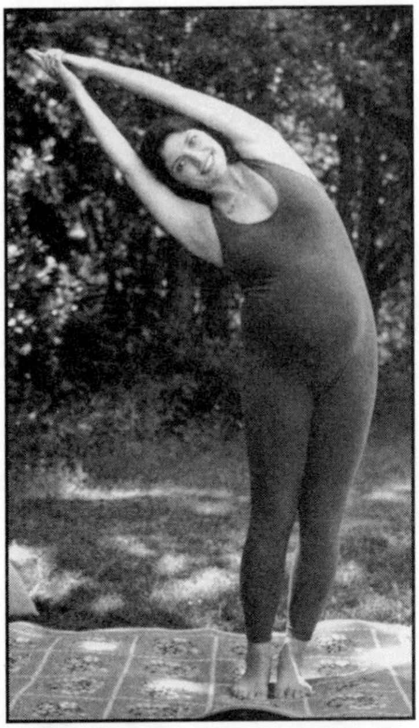

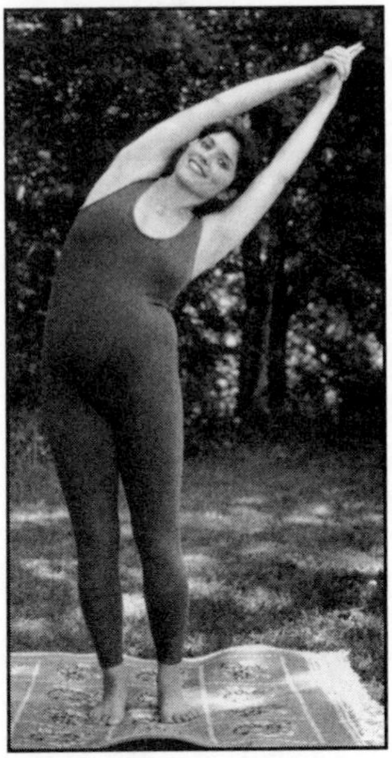

Position four: bend to the left.

Position five: step out to the right, bend your knees and your arms at the elbows for goddess pose.

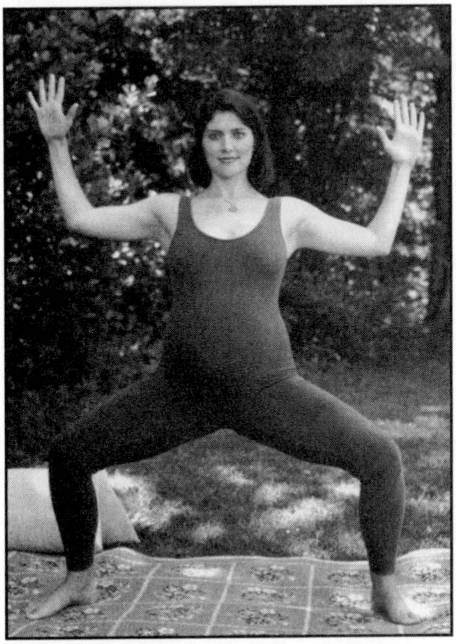

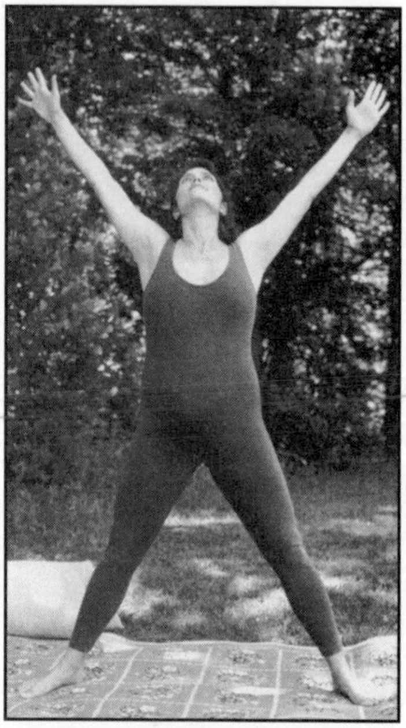

Position six: star pose.

Position seven: goddess pose.

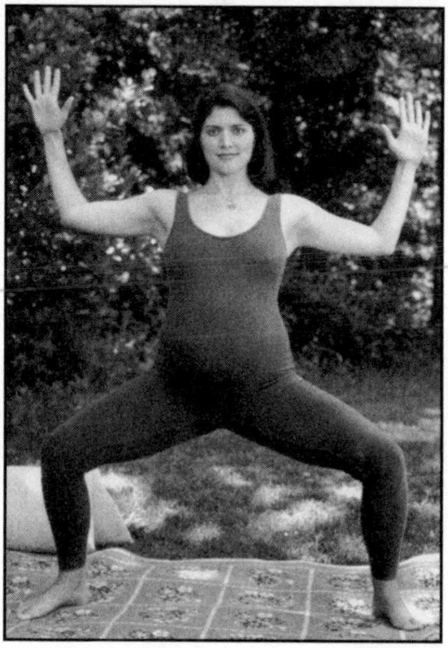

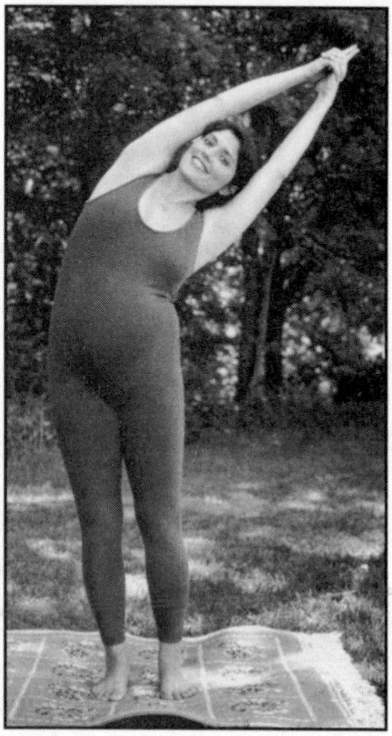

Position eight: bend to the left.

Position nine: bend to the right.

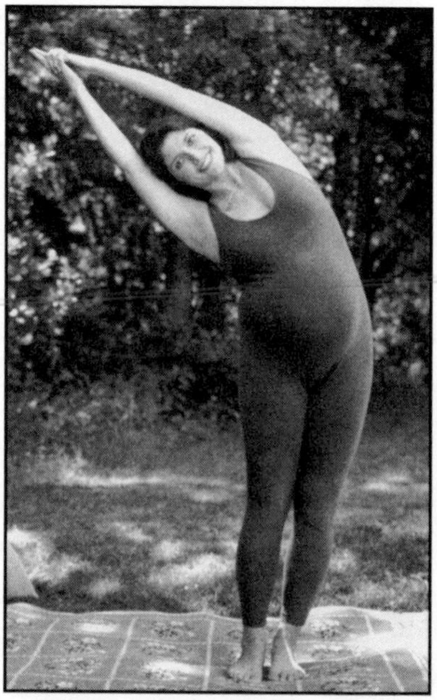

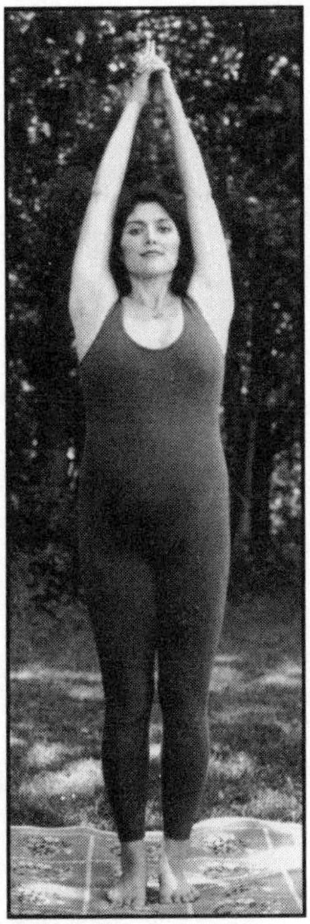

Position eleven: arms above head in steeple pose.

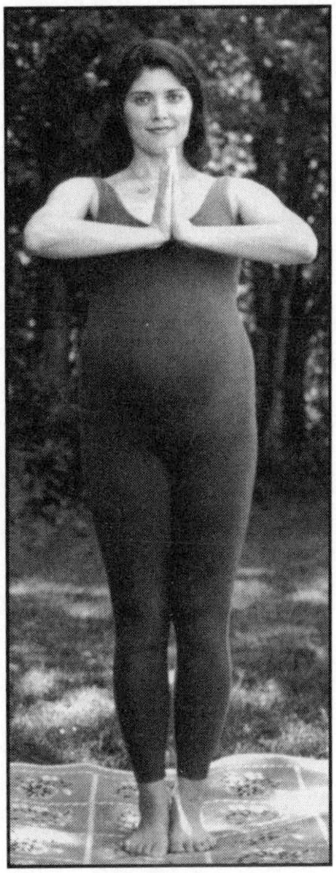

Position twelve: hands in prayer mode at the chest.

BENEFITS: The moon sequence provides a quick pick-me-up and can be done any time you want to feel rejuvenated. It stretches and strengthens the muscles of the legs, buttocks, and arms, and those that run down both sides of the body.

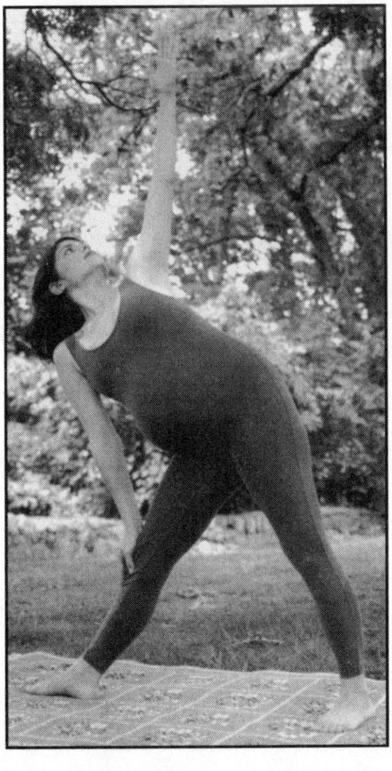

Supported Triangle: With your feet still in the wide stance of the moon sequence, turn your toes facing out at a forty-five degree angle. Inhale, then as you exhale, bend to the right, sliding your right hand down your right leg to stop just above the knee. Brace yourself with your hand on your knee for balance, and stretch your left arm up and then over, giving a stretch to your left side. Hold for fifteen to twenty seconds. Inhale and lift back to center. Repeat to the other side.

BENEFITS**:** The triangle strengthens and stretches the sides of the body and the legs. It opens up the lower back helping to reduce lower back pain and the pain of sciatica.

Inverted Pose: You will need a few pillows to do this exercise. Take your pillows and place them next to a wall (or, as shown in the picture, next to a tree) about a foot away. In this pose, do nothing but relax and breathe; however, getting into it is a little tricky. Sit on your knees in the diamond pose, with your left side next to the wall or tree, the pillows behind you. "Walk" down with your hands until you are lying on your left side. Roll over onto your back, onto the pillows. Placing your feet against the wall or tree, adjust the pillows beneath your buttocks, making them comfortable. Rest your arms at your sides or across your abdomen. Stay in this position for two to three minutes, or more if you like. Breathe deeply and relax.

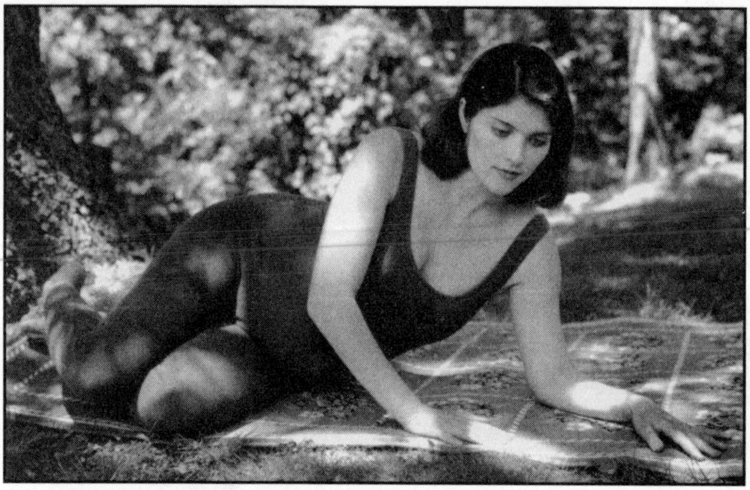

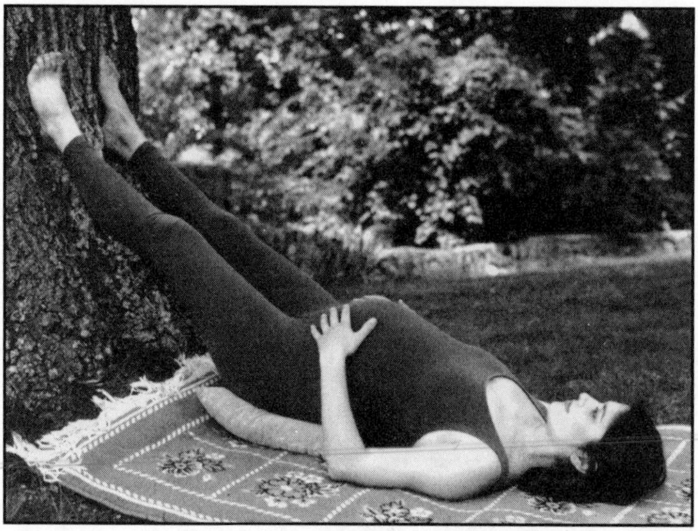

This position offers you an excellent opportunity to connect with your baby. You can use your breath to send energy to your baby. All the energy that would usually go to your legs is being centered on your mid-section. Take advantage of this. On your in-breath feel the energy coming into your body, centering on your abdomen, feel it swirling and moving in your abdomen. Don't be surprised if the baby starts to move while you are in this position. The extra blood will have energized the baby as well. Focus on your little one; feel the beneficial life energy bathing your baby in light and warmth. It is nice to leave your hands on your abdomen while you do this. It brings the energy even more into focus on your belly and when the baby moves, you can feel it. Relax every muscle in your body; forget everything, except the energy flowing in from your breath and filling your abdomen.

Doing this exercise, you are coming into contact with your baby; you may have sudden flashes about what your baby is like. Those flashes are your baby speaking to you on a telepathic level, letting you know in advance who you're carrying inside you. Relax deeply and listen. Connect with your little person. This is a good time to tell your baby anything you want it to know.

For example, during my fourth pregnancy, I was so tired and busy that I often felt guilty that the baby I carried received so little focus from me. Having had three children already, I felt ambivalent about being pregnant again, when I had so little time for myself. So I explained this to my baby. I let her know I loved her and welcomed her, and I apologized for feeling ambivalent and not having any time. Doing this eased the guilt I was feeling and created a loving flow of energy with the baby.

When you are ready to come out of the inverted pose, move slowly; bring your legs down, bending your knees, roll onto your left side, off the pillows, and walk yourself back up onto your folded knees. Stay there for a minute allowing the blood flow to readjust.

BENEFITS: No other position is better for helping the varicose veins and swollen ankles that can come with the increased amount of blood in your body during pregnancy. With the legs raised above your head, the blood flow is redirected out of the feet and legs and back into the torso.

This completes the exercise portion of the class. We now move on to the deep relaxation.

chapter 13

Deep Relaxation

The idea of doing the deep relaxation exercise is to relax completely. This is done through a systematic tensing and releasing of the individual parts of the body. By the time you have completed this process, every part of you should feel relaxed. Be aware of this goal as you follow the steps. Choosing a quiet place to do this exercise and turning down the lights or closing the curtains will help make it easier for you to forget everything else, and allow your mind, as well as your body, to sink into a deep, relaxed state.

Deep relaxation should always be done at the end of each yoga class as it helps to relieve any tension that may have built up during the class and offers a set opportunity for your body to rejuvenate.

PLACE AND POSITION: You can do this exercise anywhere that is comfortable for you—on the floor with a lot of pillows, or on the bed with a lot of pillows, or on a couch with a lot of pillows. The pillows will help you to be comfortable and allow

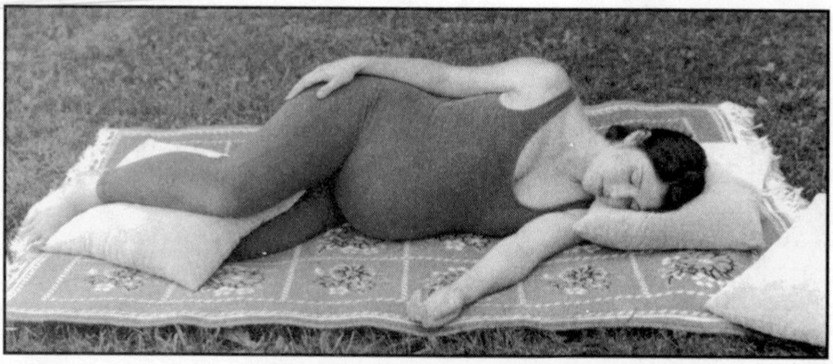

you to relax fully. The relaxation is always done on the left side as this allows for the easiest flow of maternal blood to the placenta and back again, benefiting the baby.

Lying on your left side, put one pillow under your head, another one or two under your right, top leg, which should cross over the bottom one and rest on the bed/floor/couch in front of you. Another pillow can be placed under your belly, to support its weight, if that is comfortable for you. Check to make sure that everything is supported and comfortable.

PROCEDURE: Begin with the breath: take a slow deep breath, filling the abdomen, inhaling as much as you can. Exhaling, think to yourself "relax." Inhale into the abdomen, exhale, and relax. Do this one more time: inhale, exhale, relax. On the inhale, imagine you are breathing in fresh, pure air. Inhale fresh, pure air; allow it to go to all the cells in your body to rout out any tension; exhale, and expel that tension. Inhale fresh, pure air; exhale hot, tense air. Do this a few times until you feel the tension easing.

In this exercise, you will be systematically tensing and relaxing every part of your body. Bring your awareness to your legs. Tense them. Squeeze the muscles in the legs, point the toes, tense the feet and ankles, the calves and thighs; squeeze tightly, then let all the tension go at once. Gently roll the legs a little, making them comfortable, then forget about them.

Next, bring your awareness to your buttocks. Inhaling, squeeze the buttock muscles, make them tight; inhale deeply, relax, let your breath go; relax the muscles, then forget about them.

Stretch out your arms, wiggling the fingers, rolling the wrists. Then squeeze them tight, make fists, tighten all of the muscles of the arms; squeeze and then relax, letting them fall down. Roll them a little to make sure they are comfortable, then forget about them.

Bring your awareness to your abdomen. Take a deep inhalation, push out your abdomen, fill it up, and hold the breath for a moment. When you exhale this time, let your breath burst out of your mouth. Let your stomach relax, then forget about it.

Moving to your chest, take another deep breath, inhaling into your chest. Fill it as much as possible. Hold the breath for a moment, then relax, letting the air burst out of your mouth.

Now, tense your neck and shoulders, raising your head a little, and hunch your shoulders to your ears to make them tight; squeeze and relax. Let all the tension leave your neck and shoulders; move a little to adjust your position, then forget about your neck and shoulders.

Next, squeeze your face, making a tight prune face; hold this for a moment; squeeze, then relax. Wiggle your face a little until it feels comfortable, then forget about it.

Now you will be going back over your body, part by part, checking to make sure every part is relaxed. Feel this as if a wave of relaxation is moving over your body, relaxing it completely.

Beginning with your feet, relax the toes, the soles of your feet, the heels, the tops of your feet. Relax your ankles, your calves, your knees, the fronts and backs of your thighs. Relax your buttocks, your abdomen, your lower and upper back. Relax your fingers, your wrists, your forearms, your upper arms, your shoulders. Relax your neck, your ears, the sides of your head, the back of your head, your face, the top of your head. Allow the last little bit of tension to go out through the crown of your head.

Now you will be completely relaxed, with no tension anywhere, allowing your breath to flow gently in and out.

While in this relaxed state, you can do a visualization. Imagine as you inhale that your breath brings pure energy into your body. Feel it filling you, from your head to your toes, then feel it encompassing your baby. Feel the breath turning into golden light, coming in, swirling down and cascading over your abdomen. See it enveloping your baby with light, filling it with peace and the warmth of your love. Connect with your baby, extending the deep relaxation you feel to your little one. Rest there for a moment in that peace, quiet, and love.

After a few minutes, allow your awareness to come to your mind. See how calm your mind is, how peaceful. If there are any thoughts, just watch them; become a witness watching your thoughts like clouds moving across the sky. Don't be affected by them; just watch them. As you relax more fully, you will begin to sink into a deeper relaxed state, becoming aware of a peaceful, pure energy that is beyond the mind. When you become aware of that, just rest there; rest in that peaceful state. This is the true you. Beyond the body, beyond the mind, this peaceful, clear energy is *you*. Stay there for a while, feeling it, resting in your peaceful state. (Rest here for as long as you like; at least five minutes is recommended.)

When you are ready to come out of the relaxation, bring your awareness back to the breath. Slowly begin to deepen the breathing. On each inhalation, feel fresh, pure energy flowing into you, filling every part of your body. Breathe in and feel the energy come in through the top of your head; allow it to move slowly over you, down your body, to your toes. Feel the energy revitalize you. Slowly begin to move, wiggling your fingers and toes, gently moving your arms and legs. When you are ready, sit up slowly, coming into a cross-legged position. Feel the peace and the energy that is still with you. Close your eyes and stay in that peace. Sit for a moment, enjoying the peace and stillness.

Now you have completed the relaxation. Try to do it as often as you can. If you can't make it every day, aim for three or four times a week. Even doing it once a week will bring you benefits, but doing it more will bring you more.

BENEFITS: Deep relaxation is so important that it should not be omitted. If you find you are short on time or energy, skip the exercises in the previous chapter and do only the relaxation. Learning this technique of relaxation will be invaluable to you both during the labor and delivery and for the six-week adjustment period following the baby's birth, when your energy reserves will be taxed and you could suffer from sleep deprivation.

Learning to relax deeply will help you during your labor. Relaxing during the contractions will allow your uterus to do its job of opening the cervix faster and with less difficulty.

Relaxing between the contractions will allow you to get some needed rest so your energy level will remain constant. After the baby is born, relaxation is vital due to the heavy demands, both physical and emotional, of having a new baby. Learning to rest when your baby is resting, to relax while the baby is breast-feeding, and to breathe deeply and fully, will help prevent you from getting overwhelmed.

A nice way to do this exercise is to have someone read it to you. Or you could tape-record yourself reading it then play it back.

chapter 14

Breathing Techniques

Breath, essential for life, is very often taken for granted. You can live without food for a few weeks, without water for a few days, without breath, not even for a few minutes–such is the power of breath.

Breathing is necessary in order to live, but how we breathe can also affect how we feel. Often, we can alter the way we feel by changing the way we breathe. When upset or anxious, a few deep breaths have the power to calm us. When tired, the same deep breathing can be energizing.

The following two breathing techniques can be practiced any time but are especially beneficial during pregnancy and birth.

Three-Part Breath: This is a very specific, deliberate way of breathing that allows you to take in the maximum amount of air. Begin by exhaling, fully pushing your belly in to push all the air completely out. As you inhale, let the air come into your belly first, so it pushes out like a balloon. Continuing to inhale, let the air then move up to expand your rib cage. Inhaling even more, allow the air to fill your chest, fully culminating in the lifting of your collarbones. Once you have taken in all the air you can, begin by first exhaling the air from your chest, feeling your collarbones drop and your chest contract. Next feel your rib cage contract as you push the air out of your rib cage. Lastly push the air out of your belly as you exhale fully. Inhale again into your belly, moving up to your

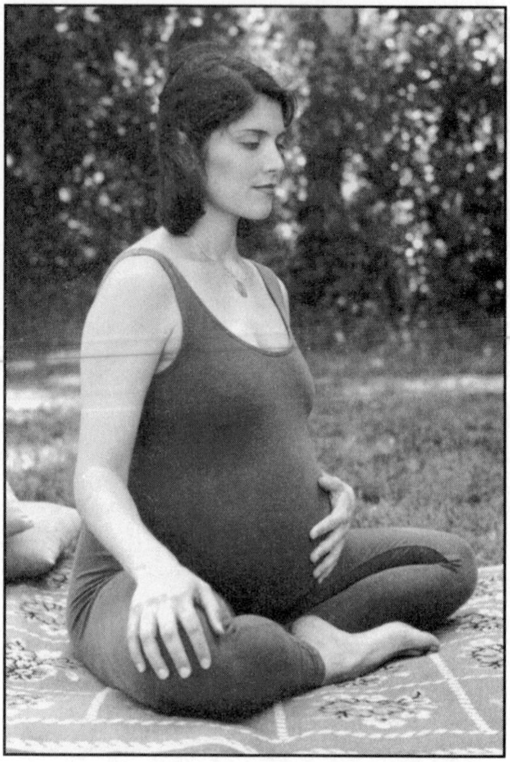

rib cage, then up into your chest. Exhale out of your chest, out of your rib cage and last, your belly comes in, pushing all of the air out. Begin by doing three full breaths in and out and move up to doing as many as you like. It is not uncommon for me to sit for fifteen or twenty minutes doing this deep three-part breathing.

BENEFITS: This breath is very relaxing and energizing. In the same way that a regular deep breath triggers the release of a chemical into your brain that makes you feel more relaxed, the depth of this breath has the same effect. With practice, this type of breath will allow you to take in enough air to fill your lungs to their capacity. This is why the breath is so energizing.

I used this breath extensively during my pregnancies to relax and rejuvenate, and during all of my births. In between contractions, it helped me to relax; during the contractions, it helped me to focus and to breathe through the pain. A variation of this breath that I also used extensively during my births is belly breathing.

Belly Breathing: Begin this breath by exhaling fully, blowing all of the air out. Breathing in, you allow the air to come in and push your belly out just as you would in the first step of three-part breathing. Inhale deeply and fully. This will cause your belly to be pushed way out. Exhale pushing out all the air, then repeat three to five times to get used to how it feels.

BENEFITS: When you have fully inhaled you will notice that your pelvic floor feels very relaxed and open. As you continue to breathe, you will notice it is almost impossible to retain a tight pelvic floor while you are belly breathing. Because of this, belly breathing is ideal to use during the dilation stage of your labor when your cervix is opening, as having a relaxed pelvic floor can facilitate the cervix opening.

This completes the sequence of exercises and relaxation and breathing techniques. It should have taken you about thirty-five to forty minutes to complete the class as presented in the last three chapters. Once you have finished, you may sit for a moment, enjoying the serenity produced by your yoga practice. Done regularly, yoga will help you have a happier and healthier pregnancy and an easier delivery.

chapter 15

Following Your Instincts

As in all things, it helps to practice a technique before you are required to depend upon it. Following your instincts is one of these techniques. God-given, like breathing, it can nevertheless require a focused effort to relearn it.

From as early as the first labor contraction, your body and mind will begin prompting you about what will help you through your birth process. This prompting may appear in the form of a simple desire, such as, wanting to have only family and close friends around you. It may be felt as a gut instinct; you may feel a strong inclination to walk, squat, moan, or to sway through a contraction. Or it may come in the form of a violent reaction against something; you may suddenly have a strong aversion to noise, bright lights, music, or conversation of any kind. All these feelings are a natural part of the birth process. They are your body's way of telling you what you need in order to have an easier and more productive labor and delivery. When listened to, this innate instinctual ability will allow you to move through your birth feeling powerful, connected to a deep inner strength.

Instinctual cues are always present, even when you are not in labor. However, they are often so subtle, you don't initially recognize them for what they are. It can help in discerning your instincts to think of them as a quiet voice, accompanied by a strong feeling; sensations you get in your heart, your gut, or your bones where you know something is so without having to think about it. Very often when you do think about it, your mind says, "That can't be so." But in your heart, you know it is.

During pregnancy, this quiet voice often grows louder. So much of your energy is occupied with making the baby that your ability for cognitive thought can be diminished, leaving an internal environment ripe for following your instincts. As the pregnancy progresses and the baby grows, you may notice you are clumsier and more forgetful than you ever have been. You may also notice you have become highly intuitive, more in touch with your feelings and with those of the people around you, resulting in a sort of second knowledge. During pregnancy, do not be surprised if you habitually know who is on the phone before you answer it, if you have a feeling your mother is coming for a visit just before she arrives, or if you can sense the feelings of other people so completely, it is almost as if they were your own.

This change in perception, though frequently viewed as making you less able to handle your life, is actually the result of a normal physiological process that prepares you for the challenges of pregnancy and delivery. Being more open and more perceptive during pregnancy contributes to your ability to bond with your baby. During birth, it allows for a more direct access to the innate knowledge that will guide and strengthen you.

During birth, your feelings and your awareness—your instincts—will guide you every step of the way. They enabled me to give birth to five children naturally, and to be able to feel good about those experiences. I knew in my heart, and in my gut, that I wanted to have my babies at home, and I knew that the use of water during labor and delivery would help my process. To know what is good for you will require your becoming quiet enough to tune in and listen. If you listen carefully, will know where you will feel most comfortable giving birth, how you will feel most comfortable, and who you will feel most comfortable having around while you do.

There are many good techniques to quiet your mind and to get in touch with your instincts. The two I have found to be most effective in my life are the "Time-out" exercise and "Free Movement Dancing."

chapter 16

Time-Out

This highly effective way to become aware of your instincts requires you take ten minutes out of your busy day to relax, unburden, ask questions of yourself, and find strength. I know the notion of finding ten minutes to be by yourself is asking a lot, but the benefits of this exercise both for pregnancy and in anticipation of birth make it worth the effort.

With five children, a house to run, a job to maintain, and a marriage to participate in, I still find time to do this simple relaxation exercise. It is invaluable. It keeps me in touch with that inner guidance system that, having led me through five births, continues to help me with raising the children. Bringing a sense of peace and space in a world where there isn't much, this simple exercise can refresh and rejuvenate you in the process of reconnecting you with your instincts.

This exercise is done in three parts. The first part is unburdening yourself of all of your worries, thereby freeing up your mind for the second part; the second part is asking yourself pertinent questions; leading to the third part which is finding your inner strength.

To practice this exercise, find a place that is as quiet as possible, preferably one where you won't be disturbed. Sometimes the only quiet place in my house is the bathroom, so that's where I go. When I do this, I tell my children I am putting myself in "time-out," hence, the name. They love this and are surprisingly understanding. As I am all too often stressed to the maximum and storming around the house, practicing this "time-out" exercise gives me a much-needed break, and gives the children a chance to be the understanding ones.

Take a position, either sitting or standing, that is as comfortable as possible so you will be able to fully relax. Sitting in a comfortable chair may work well; sometimes lying down will work better. My favorite non-pregnancy position for this exercise is the yoga position called the *Savasana* or "corpse" pose. This is done by lying flat on your back on the bed or floor; your legs about shoulder-width apart; your arms straight out at your sides a little away from your body; your palms turned up. This position is very relaxing as it eases the tension in your neck in a way sitting doesn't. This position is good for the first trimester; the second and third trimester pregnancy require a modification of this pose as it is not recommended for women after their third month to lie on their backs for more than a few minutes. The position for later pregnancy is the one done during the deep relaxation exercise of the yoga class. Accomplish it by lying on your left side with a pillow under your head and another one under your right knee that lays slightly across the bottom of the left leg. More pillows can be used anywhere you need them to make yourself comfortable.

Once you have established your place and position, it is time to begin. The first part is the "breath unburden mode." For this part of the exercise, you may use the three-part breathing technique described in the yoga class, or you may use simple deep breathing. Begin by exhaling fully, then slowly allow the air to come back in. Do three slow, deep breaths. Even just these three, slow breaths will have an effect on you. Tension ebbs, worries recede.

After you have done three plain breaths, begin to unburden. On each exhalation, unload all of your worries, on each inhalation, replace them with a new thought. Exhale: "I am exhaling Jimmy hitting the baby over the head with the Power Ranger." Inhale: "I am inhaling this quiet moment for myself." Exhale: "I am exhaling the person in the car who yelled at me for cutting them off on the freeway." Inhale: "I inhale total love and forgiveness." Exhale: "I am exhaling my inability to concentrate on the work I brought home from the office." Inhale: "I inhale peace and clarity."

Exhale whatever is bothering you and replace it with something better. If you can't always think of a new, better thing to inhale, pick one inhalation "topic" that means a lot to you and repeat that every time. Here are a few general suggestions: "I inhale total peace and acceptance." "I inhale contentment and clarity."

Do as many of these breaths as you need to begin feeling peaceful and relaxed, taking perhaps five minutes or so. Let all of your worries go, and give yourself fully to this process of unburdening.

After you complete the unburdening, let your breathing return to normal. Remain still for a minute, enjoying the cessation of mental activity that comes from unloading all of your worries. It's amazing how just taking a moment out of your day to consciously address and let go of what has been bothering you can make you feel so much more relaxed.

In this relaxed state, with your mind so still and calm, begin to ask yourself questions. This is the time to think about your birth and to ask yourself how you would like it to be. This is also the time to begin addressing any fears you might have. In this quiet state, consider you fears. Do they come from doubts about your ability, or ignorance of the birth process? Have other people been telling you how terrible their births were? What are the origins of your fears? Try to distinguish between what is making you feel afraid, and what is making you feel warned. Listen closely. If it is fear that is talking, remind yourself that birth is natural and normal, and not something that you need to fear. Remind yourself that you are preparing mentally, physically, and emotionally now, to be able to go through this process. You do not need to be afraid of birth, but you do need to listen closely. An inner urging that may appear as fear, may instead be your instincts telling you something.

I am one of six children, five of whom were born naturally, none of whom were born at home. My mother had always been interested in home birth, but never had access to it until her last baby. When she became pregnant for the sixth time at age thirty-seven, we had a doctor and a midwife in our community who were both capable and willing to attend home births. It appeared that my mother's chance for a home birth had come. She and my father were very excited, anticipating the new addition and this new experience of birth.

A couple of months into the pregnancy, however, my mother begin to have misgivings; she had a deep sense she would be better off in the hospital. She discussed this with her doctor who said she was certainly healthy enough to have the baby at home, but that it was very important for her to feel completely comfortable with the decision. She recommended my mother spend some quiet time considering both options. Each time my mother would consider these options she would feel resistance to the idea of giving birth at home even though, theoretically and philosophically, she agreed with home birth. From this "sense" she made her decision to go to the hospital. Once made, she felt very comfortable with her decision.

When my sister was born, she had a condition that required she be in the Intensive Care Unit for three days. One of her lungs wasn't working, and her blood sugar level was so low, she nearly didn't make it. Immediate medical intervention was the only way she was able to survive.

I have told you this story not to add one more "horror" story to the database illustrating how scary birth can be. I've told you this so you will understand the importance of listening to and following your instincts, even when they don't agree with what you philosophically believe. By listening carefully, you will know long before your birth what environment is right for you, who you would like to be present, and what "props" or "aids" you would like to have available at your birth, all by asking yourself these questions and then waiting for the quiet responses.

I knew home birth was right for me, without a doubt in my mind. Waterbirth was the same way; I just knew that it was the ideal environment for me to birth in. Tuning in to your instincts should allow you to make the choice that is right for you. Be open to everything, and do what you feel the most comfortable with.

After you have done the Time-Out exercise a few times to become familiar with it, you can even bring a pen and paper to your quiet space. As you ask yourself questions, write the answers down. This way you will have it written exactly as it was answered, without having to try to remember it.

The last part of this exercise is to create something new. You have already unburdened yourself of all the things that were bothering you, and you have spent some time asking questions, learning about what is important to you. Now, take advantage of this focused time to create.

Think of how you would like your birth to be. Imagine peace and serenity, power and quiet confidence. Imagine and feel that you are fully able to birth your baby. Dwell on the feeling of being capable and all-powerful. This is where your strength is: in knowing and believing that you *can* do it. The strength and confidence that you feel now will be there for you during birth. Get used to this feeling. During your birth, everything else around you will serve only to remind you of this quiet strength. The strength itself is yours.

The more you do this exercise, the easier it will become to release what is bothering you, to get in touch with your instincts, and to remind yourself where your strength lies. From practicing this often, the sensation of inner knowledge and confidence will begin to permeate your life, becoming familiar and readily available to you once labor commences and your baby is on the way.

chapter 17

Free Movement Dance

Movement is very helpful during pregnancy, not only in keeping you fit, but also in keeping you in touch with your instincts. Often your body will react instinctually without your mind even being aware of it, making movement an effective way to tap into your instincts. Movement is also an important aspect of feeling powerful during your birth, making feeling free to move an important thing to become familiar with in anticipation of your birth.

One simple, effective way of establishing a connection with your instinctual self and becoming familiar with moving instinctually is through "Free Movement Dance."

Pick some music, anything you like, but make it something that inspires you to move. As the music plays, begin by centering yourself, standing firmly on both feet, your posture erect, your arms hanging loose at your sides. Sway slowly back and forth a few times, loosening everything up. Do a few neck and shoulder rolls, arm circles, and wrist rotations.

Then begin "moving." Not a specific form of movement; the idea is not necessarily to "dance," but simply to move, without focus or form, just feeling your body. Pay attention to each part individually. How does your arm feel? Where is it tight? Where is it loose? What parts are weak? What parts are strong? Is there specific tension anywhere? Lift your arm, rotate it, do whatever "feels" best, whatever you feel inclined to do.

Pay attention to each part of your body as you move, and then consider your body as a whole. During pregnancy, when your rapidly changing body can feel so foreign, this type of simple movement allows you to note the changes that are taking place, leading to an easier acceptance of those changes. If you get a Braxton-Hicks contraction during this exercise (intermittent painless uterine contractions occuring every ten to twenty minutes), as you often will during movement, use it to experiment with what positions feel best during the contraction; try squatting, or leaning over a chair. Once it goes, experiment to see what will allow you to release your tension more readily. Take a few deep breaths, shake out your arms, wiggle your legs, roll your hips around a few times. Get used to how it feels to release your tension, as well as how best to go through the tension of the contractions.

Your Free Movement Dance exercise can be as long, or as short, as you like. This exercise is not specifically for fitness, though that will be a side benefit. After you are through, be sure to move more slowly, cooling down, taking a few minutes to allow your breathing and your heart rate to return to normal.

chapter 18

The Perfect Place

The environment in which you decide to give birth will ideally be supportive of your natural inclination for peace, quiet, warmth, darkness, and familiarity. In this kind of environment, where you feel safe and secure, it will be easier for you to relax and let your baby be born.

If you have decided to give birth in your own home, it is likely that you already have this type of environment, and a few, simple touches will only add to the peaceful atmosphere. In a hospital or birth center, the same things that are used to make a home birth environment better, can be used to recreate the peace and familiarity you would feel at home.

TOPICAL HELPERS: There are many things that will make it easier for you to labor and deliver by helping you relax and feel more comfortable during your birth. Being able to be in a tub of water is one of these things. If you don't have a tub available, water can still be a soothing addition. Many women find standing in a hot shower with the water running over them, massaging their backs, very relaxing. Making sure not to slip, you may even squat, or labor on all fours while in the shower. Cool compresses applied to the back of the neck and the face can also help, as can other "topical" applications, such as massage.

Having a massage therapist available during labor will not only keep your muscles relaxed but can also help to keep the birthing attendants in the proper state of comfort. You will be very sensitive to the vibrations of the people around you and will find it more difficult to relax if they are tense or stressed. Massage will help them to remain in a relaxed state, better able to be there for you.

A massage therapist can help you by providing counter pressure to your lower back and massaging your legs during the contractions. This will help to keep you from tensing these areas up. Having your feet massaged is also relaxing, providing an alternate focus while you labor. Your one consideration if you are having a waterbirth is to be sure to wipe off any excess massage oil before entering the tub.

MUSIC: Choose a piece or two of music early on in your pregnancy that really resonates with you, making you feel relaxed or inspired. Then begin using that piece of music anytime you are going to take time out to relax. Doing this will create a positive association with that particular piece of music, meaning that every time you hear it, you will relax automatically. You might also like to include the music you use for the Free Movement Dance exercise. This music may work better for the earlier, or more active, phases of labor where moving freely helps. Later on, your more relaxing choice of music may be played to help you to relax deeply.

AROMATHERAPY: A simple, yet very effective way to alter your environment is through the use of scent, achieved by burning incense or the use of essential oils. In the same way that a certain piece of music becomes associated with a certain response, scents also possess the ability to alter your mood. If you use incense, select one that appeals to you and burn it any time you are taking time out to consciously relax. Then, when you burn it during labor, it will act just like the music, easing your ability to relax.

If you use essential oils to alter your mood, you will have the added benefit of their being theraputic as well as pleasant smelling. Rose, geranium, neroli, and lavender are all safe oils to use, and each provides its own benefit.

Rose is a good cardiac tonic, a natural antiseptic, and has a slightly analgesic effect, which makes it a nice addition to a massage oil, and its scent is pleasant and not overpowering.

Geranium is highly effective in improving circulation. It is specifically good for the uterus, and the whole female reproductive system, and is known for its anti-depressant effect.

Neroli, produced from the fresh flowers of the bitter orange tree, is beneficial to the nervous system, and promotes easy breathing. It has a sedating and calming effect, and helps to improve the circulation.

Lavender stimulates the circulation and is calming and slightly analgesic. Its pleasant, slightly spicy aroma is well tolerated by nearly everyone, which makes this a good choice if you are unfamiliar with essential oils.

Essential oils are used by either placing a few drops in boiling water to allow the steam to carry them into the air, or by using an aromatherapy pot, designed specifically for use with essential oils. You can get an aromatherapy pot at your local health food store.

LIGHTING: Placing candles around the room and lowering the lights, if you are able, will make whatever room you are in more inviting during labor. In your highly sensitized state, bright lights may seem glaring, causing you to become anxious and tense. Lowering the existing lighting as much as you can will provide a feeling of quietness and comfort. Lighting a few candles will soften the light even further. A lighted candle will also provide you with a good point of focus that you can use to keep yourself centered during intense contractions.

FAMILY AND FRIENDS: Deciding who to have at your birth is an important decision to make, as every person who is in the room with you will have an effect on your energy during the labor and delivery. In labor, you are likely to be very sensitive to the feelings and vibrations of the people around you. This is why some studies have shown that having a person present to specifically provide support for the woman in labor can cause her labor to be shorter, with fewer complications.

Think carefully about who you want to have with you during your birth. Select only those people you feel truly comfortable with and who you feel will provide the most support to you during your labor. My midwife, my husband, and both of my parents were always present during my births. This was a good "team" for me. I felt comfortable with every person present, and they, in turn, provided me with the support and encouragement I needed as I progressed through my labors.

Other considerations for the birth environment are to keep lots of beverages on hand to keep you well hydrated. I drank Recharge during my births; this is a natural juice rich in electrolytes that can be found at health food stores. In the hospital you may not be allowed to eat or drink during your labor. An IV will be used to keep you from becoming dehydrated.

Have light snacks available, such as fresh fruits, vegetable soups, yogurt, or anything else that is simple and easy to digest. These snacks will help you keep your strength up, as well as that of your partner or birth attendants. Your appetite is likely to be unpredictable during labor. You may want something completely different from what is suggested here. Bring and eat what you think you will want. After the baby is born, you are likely to be ravenous, particularly for carbohydrates. After the birth of each of my babies, I ate my mother's potato soup and crackers. Nothing tasted better to me, nor replenished my energy quicker. Try to imagine what you would like and have that on hand.

All of the "aids" that I have outlined here are only suggestions to provide you with an idea of what you may want during your birth event. None of them are required for you to have a positive birth experience. How you feel about birth and your ability to give birth are much more important than where you give birth, and what and who you have around you while you do. Taking care of that should be your most important consideration.

Part III

The Practice

chapter 19

Birth Stories

For my four home births, I had midwife Mary Carmichael, attend me. In addition to her, my husband, Nilakantan, and my parents, Bhagavan and Bhavani, were there. With my family's support and Mary's gentle guidance, I was able to give birth to my babies naturally.

It was nice that way because no one told me what to do or how to do it. Instead they encouraged me to do whatever I felt like doing, such as walking around in the wet grass in my bare feet, listening to the patter of rain on the leaves.

My fifth baby was born in a birth center, and I found this to be a new experience. Unable to depend on my surroundings for familiarity and support, I turned to that which was the most familiar in my births: the water. Through its warmth and closeness, I was able to relax and give birth to my fifth child.

All five of my births progressed smoothly and uneventfully. At each moment I was aware of what was going on, both inside me and around me. Laboring and delivering in my home, I felt relaxed and comfortable. There was no chaos or nervousness to deal with, and no one to tell me I wasn't proceeding within the "normal" limits.

Birthing in this way was freeing and empowering. Trusting myself to be able to give birth gave me the confidence to trust in myself, and in my ability as a mother. As birthing came naturally, so mothering came naturally. Not easily, necessarily: there are many challenges in life, and giving birth is only one of them. But without interference or hindrance, the babies naturally just came. For me, giving birth became a part of the joy of having children instead of a traumatic ordeal that had to be gone through in order to get children.

By sharing these experiences of giving birth naturally, I hope to give women a different view of what birth can be. I hope that by reading this, you may find it within yourselves to embrace this experience of giving birth more fully, of believing in yourselves and in the miracle of your babies and the greatness and wisdom of creation.

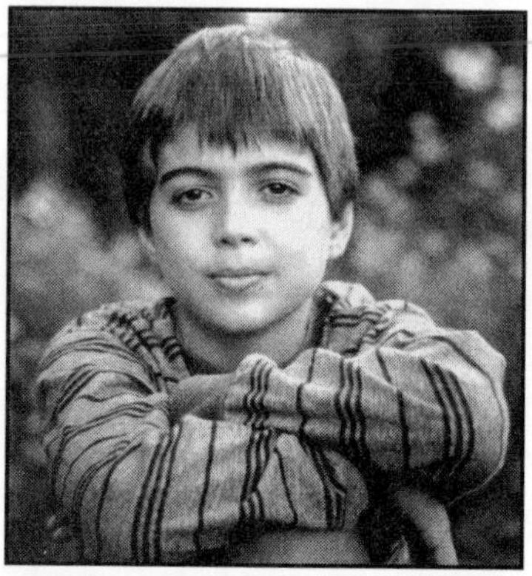

chapter 20

My First Water Baby

Sampath Moses, born March 29, 1988, 4:07 A.M., twenty-two and a half inches long, weighing eight pounds, fourteen ounces.

My first baby was preceded by weeks of anticipation. With this being my first, and I being not a patient person, I spent the entire last month of my pregnancy either getting things ready for the baby's birth, or trying to occupy myself with other things in order to forget about the baby's impending birth.

Finding out about waterbirth the week I was due was a wonderful distraction. I had plenty to read and plenty to do to help me forget that a baby could be born any day. So, when I woke up on the morning of March 28, feeling the practice contractions called Braxton-Hicks contractions that had become my regular companions over the last three weeks, I wondered, again, if today was to be the day.

March 28, 1988:

It is a beautiful, cold spring morning. Too cold yet for many flowers to have pushed their dainty heads above the surface; only the crocuses are brave enough and they sit bright-colored against the dark earth.

I am one day overdue, and having the usual Braxton-Hicks. I wake early and yawn, stretching, wondering, once again, "Will today be the day?"

On my way through the living room/kitchen area to the bathroom, I pass by the birthing tub. I smile when I see it sitting on the linoleum where it meets the carpet. A few feet away on the living room floor sits a couch cushion; another leans against the wall behind it. They have been covered with large plastic bags and draped with a sheet. It is here that I will sit after I have given birth to my baby. Next to this is the stainless steel bowl to hold the placenta, some towels for me to dry off with when I get out of the tub, and blankets for the new baby.

I am so excited; everything is ready.

As I pass by the birthing tub, I pause and place my hands on the rim, leaning over, looking down into its two and a half foot depth. Yesterday we had our first trial run of filling it. It took one and a half hours as we had to let the water heater heat up twice. Once it was full, my husband and I got in and relaxed in the breast-deep water. It felt wonderful. Having had no bath at all, only showers, during my pregnancy, I found the water was warm, and relaxing, and soothing. After so many months during which my body weight only increased, floating in the tub made me feel nearly weightless. I slept so well last night because of how relaxed it made me feel.

I notice when I am coming back through the kitchen from the bathroom that the contraction I am having seems stronger than the others. I feel a surge of excitement but tell myself not to. Having experienced a "false" labor a week ago with similar stronger and more regular contractions, I know this could still just be my body practicing for the real thing.

Nilakantan wakes up, we have breakfast, then clean up from breakfast and I have had three contractions, about twenty to twenty-five minutes apart. I decide to call Mary, my midwife. While I wait for her to come, I pace around the house feeling nervous and excited. I am afraid she will come and tell me I am not in labor. I am so anxious for my baby to come. As I wait I think about holding my baby in my arms and automatically place my hands on my stomach to feel the jabs and wriggles. I ask the baby if it is coming today.

I feel no fear of the upcoming birth, only anticipation. I know that birth is natural and that I have the ability to birth my baby. But I do feel nervous. I have not given birth before and I wonder what it will be like.

When Mary arrives, she gives me a pelvic exam to check my cervix for dilation. It is one and one-half centimeters dilated; my contractions are still regular at twenty minutes apart. It appears my baby is coming!

As the day goes by, I take a walk in the woods. It is beautiful outside, with the first warm breath of spring making the air so fresh after the winter. When I get back from my walk I rest. My contractions are still coming, but they are not strong and I don't even think of them as being painful. I eat a light meal at lunch, but am not very hungry, and I remember to drink to keep my body hydrated.

In early evening Nilakantan leaves to go to my parents' house to wait with my father for the more active phase of labor to come. He watches *Star Trek* while I sit with Mary and Bhavani, listening to what it was like for them in giving birth to their eleven collective children, only one of whom was born at home. We laugh and talk and their stories help me to feel less nervous. I believe them when they tell me I will do fine.

By nine P.M., I feel a distinct difference in my contractions. Active labor has begun. The contractions are much stronger and harder, now. Each one begins in my lower back then radiates around to my lower abdomen, then up over my whole belly, until it is as hard as a rock. It stays that way for twenty to thirty seconds and then gradually tapers off. I notice how the pain I feel mirrors the contractions, starting in my lower back, wrapping up around my abdomen, and then it continues, shooting down my legs. These contractions hurt, but it is a strange kind of pain, very much like a large muscle cramping. Breathing deeply helps. Each deep breath pushes out my belly and relaxes my abdominal muscles. Doing this, I can remember to relax my legs, my bottom, my neck, and shoulders. During the contractions I focus on allowing my cervix to open. Focusing on the work my body is doing helps me to forget about the pain. When each contraction is over, I breathe deeply and slowly, letting go, letting everything relax.

I notice that the contractions are becoming more intense in stages. Every time I get comfortable with their intensity, the next one that comes is stronger, building in a gradual, persistent way. Through this ever-increasing rhythm, I find I am able to handle the pain, taking each contraction as it comes, and relaxing in between.

Soon though, sitting still is no longer comfortable. I find I want to move. I get up and begin walking back and forth. Mary walks with me, holding my hand and rubbing my back when I stop to breathe through a contraction. She is watching me closely; she has seen the shift in my energy to a more restless, dynamic energy as active labor takes hold. I have passed through early labor and can get into the tub whenever I like. She asks if I want it filled, and I say that I do. Nilakantan has come home and he hooks up the hose and begins to fill it.

The lights are low and a fire burns warmly in the wood stove. Six candles provide soft light. I take my nightgown off. It feels better to be naked, unhindered, free. It is quiet and warm and comforting with only candlelight flickering. Everyone speaks in hushed tones as I walk slowly back and forth stopping to breathe through the pain of each contraction, then continuing on.

I can hear the water running. The sound of it fills me with longing. I go over to the tub and look in. It has only just begun to fill. I ask when it will be ready. They tell me it will take an hour. An hour is a lifetime.

I am restless while I wait and pace back and forth, stopping with each contraction. Every few minutes I check the tub. Slowly it fills, and I can get in. By now, the contractions are strong and the pain is intense. I know the water will help. Instinctively, I know.

I step over the edge of the tub and sink down into the warm water. The water is warm and soothing. I sigh, sinking deeper. The first thing I notice is how the pain across my lower abdomen, like a tight band, is gone as is the intense pressure in my pelvis, my legs, and my lower back. I close my eyes and lay my head back on the towel someone has placed on the edge of the tub. The tension leaves me as I rest completely.

When I feel another contraction coming, I brace myself for the pain I am now used to feeling. I breathe deeper as it begins to build. It peaks and tapers off without me feeling much pain. I am amazed; it has come and gone with my hardly knowing. I sigh and lay my head back. Another contraction comes, I stir enough to breathe through it and then close my eyes and rest once again.

I feel so different laboring in the water. I feel so much less pain, I almost feel like I am cheating. I smile at that, noticing that not only has the water relaxed my body, it has soothed my mind as well. I no longer feel as if I can't do it. All uncertainty has left me. I feel strong and confident and suddenly I know this birth will be wonderful. Mary and my mother were right, I am doing fine.

Somewhere in the early hours in the morning the contractions come hard and close together. I have been in the water for a couple of hours, now, but even in the water I have little relief. Mary watches me closely. She and my mother are beside me, encouraging me. They tell me it will be soon now.

During the peak of one contraction I feel a pop inside. The membranes have ruptured. I jump from the unexpected force of it and am immediately nauseous. I begin to lean out of the tub so I don't throw up in the tub. Mary brings a bowl to the tub so I don't throw up in the water. We meet halfway when she hits me in the face with it. A second later, I am throwing up into the bowl and it seems to make the contractions even stronger.

With this intense energy, I begin to make sounds to help me through each pain. I bellow a sustained "Om" or "Ah." For a while, it feels good to do this, giving me a focus for the intense energy being generated by the contractions. And it gives me an alternative focus. Instead of focusing on the tightness and the pain of the contractions, I focus on the depth of the sound I am making.

The contractions continue, coming together closer and closer; I have little time to rest. Each one is so powerful, I can no longer stay on top of the pain. I bellow "Om" and "Ah," I breathe deep. Nothing helps.

I don't want to do it anymore; I decide I'm done, I quit. I tell everyone I don't want to do it anymore. They speak to me encouragingly. I barely hear them; all of my effort goes into getting through each contraction. I sink deep inside myself, knowing only the rhythm of labor, the contraction and the rest, and I notice that this contraction is different. At the end of it I feel an incredible urge to push. I hold my breath automatically and push hard until the urge leaves me.

I hear Mary saying, "Good, good, you're starting to push out your baby." I feel a new excitement. This energy is so powerful I begin to shake. Another contraction, I push again. I can't believe how strong this contraction is. It doesn't feel the same as before; it doesn't hurt, it is just overwhelmingly strong. I feel pressure in my lower back and bottom as I push the baby down through the pelvic bones. Another rest, I breathe deeply. I am more aware now. I note that my mother and father are there, Nilakantan is behind me, supporting me in a raised squat and encouraging me. I listen to Mary reminding me to relax and then to push hard during the contraction. She reaches down and feels for the baby. The top of the baby's head is beginning to come out. Mary tells me I can feel it if I want to.

I reach down and feel a small lump covered with soft hair. I can't believe it, the baby is right there, ready to be born. My heart goes out to the little one; I speak softly, welcoming. Another contraction and I feel burning and stinging as I push and the perineum stretches. I push the head all the way out. Mary has her hands on the baby's head, gently holding him, waiting. Another pushing contraction comes on almost immediately. I feel the baby turning slightly and the shoulders come out, then the whole baby slides out into the water. Mary has hold of the baby. She holds him under the water for a moment, making sure that the umbilical cord is not wrapped around his neck, and she feels for the sex. The baby is a boy. Mary gently lifts him out of the water and places him in my arms.

I look down into small, wide eyes that are looking around quietly. I am so surprised by how much of a person he is. He is so present and aware. Mary suctions his nose and mouth with a bulb syringe to make sure there is no water in his mouth that could be inhaled. There is no need; he has already begun to breathe on his own. I sink his body back down into the water so he can feel the warmth of it again. He looks peacefully curious as he stretches out his arms and legs, opening and relaxing in this familiar element. Around me everyone has crowded close and is speaking to him in excited whispers. Nilakantan leans in close. He reaches out and touches his hand, the small fingers close around his. I smile at him and say, "You know, I could do that again. Not immediately, necessarily, but in a few years from now, I could do it again."

And I did.

chapter 21

Birth of an Englishman

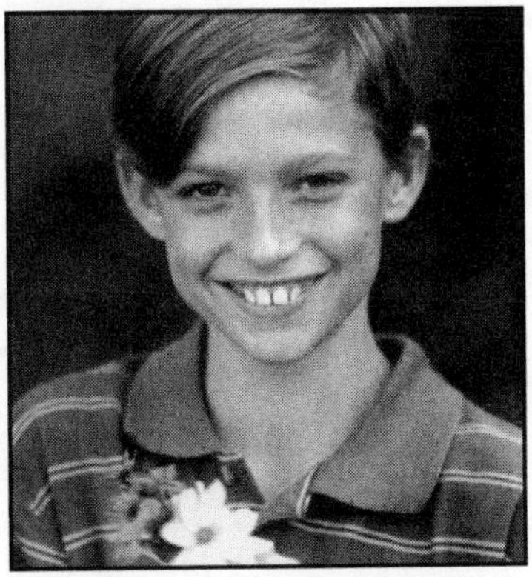

Nataraja Daniel, born March 12, 1990, 4:22 P.M., twenty-two and a half inches long, weighing nine pounds.

My second pregnancy had little of the glowing ease of my first pregnancy. I was thoroughly exhausted from running around after an eighteen-month old, and would have been perfectly happy to have gone to bed and stayed there for the duration. I lost ten pounds during the first three months from feeling nauseous and remained thin for the rest of my pregnancy, which is probably why Mary thought our baby was going to be small, only seven and a half pounds or so.

March of that year was unseasonably warm, as I anxiously awaited the new one's arrival, becoming more and more frustrated as my due date came and went with no baby.

March 12, 1990

I have not slept well in the last couple of weeks, having so many Braxton-Hicks contractions. Many more than I had during the last few weeks of my pregnancy with Sampath. Two weeks ago I thought the baby was coming for sure. My contractions were strong and regular for almost three hours. Mary came and gave me a pelvic exam. There was no dilation and only a little effacement. Clearly my baby was not on the way.

Every morning for the last eight days, since my baby was due, I have woken up tired and resigned, feeling so frustrated. I have tried everything I can think of to get my labor started. I have eaten large meals, gone for walks; I have ridden miles in a bumpy truck, to no avail. It doesn't seem to matter what I do, this baby is not ready to come.

As usual I wake up in the early hours of the morning, having contractions. I am irritated by this, I know the baby probably isn't coming, and I just want to go back to sleep. I sigh and roll over, tuck the pillow under my chin and try to sleep. Another one comes and it goes, but my lower back still aches. I tuck another pillow under my belly and try to relax the tension in my lower back. It still hurts as another contraction comes on. I sit up and I feel better. I realize the contractions seem to hurt more while I am lying down. This gives me an idea.

I grab my pillow and a blanket from the bottom of the bed and head toward the living room. On the couch, I wrap the blanket around me and tuck the pillow behind my head. I hardly feel the next contraction, and soon I am sleeping again, waking up with an occasionally harder contraction, or to change my position to keep from getting stiff. I sit sleeping propped up like this though the rest of the night.

Dawn comes with the early spring birds chirping, and the sun shining in through the window, waking me from my half-sleep. The sun is shining brightly and I wonder if it is going to be as unseasonably hot today as it was yesterday.

I think of that as I stretch and get up. Two years ago, when Sampath was born, we had to keep a roaring fire in the stove to make sure the house was warm enough for him once he was born. Yesterday it was eighty-five degrees. With the sunlight already warm on the door step, we won't need to have a fire at all. It makes me think today would be a great day to have our baby.

Nilakantan smiles at me indulgently when I tell him I am having contractions. He is used to hearing that by now. We have already had two "false" labors. He has a meeting in a town forty-five minutes away. I don't want him to go, afraid if I am in labor, he will miss the birth. It is so important to me that he be here. We decide to call Mary and ask her to come over and check me before he goes, just to make sure.

When I call her she says that even if I am in labor, Nilakantan has time to go and get back again, and so he leaves and I am by myself, tidying up the kitchen, folding the laundry, and waiting for Mary to come.

She gets here around eight-thirty A.M. I walk out onto the porch to meet her.

"So, you've finally decided to have that baby?" She smiles as she walks up the steps and hugs me.

"I sure hope so, I can't stand waiting any longer!" We walk arm-in-arm back into the house. On the couch she sits with me through a couple of contractions. Even without checking my cervix she can tell by the quality of the contractions that I am in labor. I am so relieved and all at once, I'm excited. I call my parents and tell them to cancel all their plans, we're having a baby, today! Today is their twenty-fifth wedding anniversary, so they are going to spend most of the day celebrating together, and will only come over when the birth is imminent.

This leaves Mary and me alone, which is fine this time. I feel none of the anxiety I felt during Sampath's labor; this time I know what to expect.

Inside the house is dark and cool, outside it is heating up already. By eleven the temperature is eighty degrees. My contractions have continued to come, getting irregularly but progressively stronger. Mary checks my cervix and finds that I am four centimeters dilated already. I am so surprised; I have hardly felt I was in labor, and yet I have come so far already. This news does cause us a little bit of concern as the tub is not set up or even in the house yet.

Mary and I set to work moving the furniture in the living room around to make room for the tub. Outside, we scrub and rinse out the tub. During contractions, I stop and breathe, remembering to relax. The contractions still aren't painful, but they are definitely getting stronger. Once the tub has been cleaned and put inside, Mary begins filling it. She seems to think this baby could be coming soon. Outside, I sit on the front steps and soak up the sun. I am wearing a sleeveless shirt and the sun feels wonderful on my arms and my upturned face. An hour goes by and Nilakantan returns. My labor is much stronger now, and as I go in the house, I feel a sudden, strong desire to get into the water. It is close enough to full that I can get in. I shed my clothes and step into the warm water. It relaxes me immediately and the familiarity of it gives me a boost of confidence. But I am tired by now from not sleeping well, and I progress slowly.

An hour after I enter the tub, I get out so Mary can check my progress. I have only dilated two centimeters. As she feels my cervix, she can tell that the opening is tipped way back, which means the baby's head is not pressing on it as well as it could be. She thinks the baby is probably lying with his spine alongside mine in the posterior position, which is why his head is not pressing directly on the cervix.

She suggests that I stay out of the water for a while and do a few squats to see if that will help the cervix to open more effectively. I squat through the next couple of contractions, but I am so tired, I just want to sleep. I lie down on the floor and fall instantly into deep sleep. I sleep for nearly half an hour without a contraction.

Sleeping so soundly gives me some badly needed rest and rejuvenates me. The contraction that comes next wakes me. It is so strong it gets me up off the ground and back into the tub.

My labor is strong and regular now. I remember what this is like. I breathe through each pain and relax in between, resting my head on the edge of the tub. The sun slants across the room as it goes from early to late afternoon. My contractions continue to come, hard and close together through transition. This time is difficult, just as it was with Sampath. I make loud sounds through each pain, and breathe deeply. It is over very quickly, though, as I feel the urge to push.

When I birthed Sampath, I sustained a small tear from pushing out both of his shoulders at once. Mary has warned me about this, so I can be conscious this time to go more slowly. She also warns that the baby may have to turn around into the more common anterior position with his back facing outward in order to be born, as he is lying in the posterior position, with his back facing inward, lying along my spine. This could be very painful for me, but I don't notice any difference while pushing and am surprised by how quickly his head crowns.

As in Sampath's birth, once his head appears at the opening, I reach down and touch him. His head comes out easily and I still want to push. Mary reminds me to go slowly, to stop pushing, but the urge is too powerful. I can't stop. She tells me to pant, and so I begin a light rapid breath through my mouth. It works and without a push, the baby's shoulders ease out one, and then the other.

I look down as the baby is born. The baby comes out face-up and as the arms are born, the baby reaches out to grasp the water. I reach down and take hold of the small hands; the fingers wrap tightly around mine, holding onto me. Half born and half unborn, the baby looks up through the water at me. One more push and the rest of the body is born. Mary checks for the sex: another boy. He has the umbilical cord wrapped around his neck once. She slides it over his head and then gently brings him to the surface. His face meets air, he inhales, and then wails, loud, gusting cries. After Sampath being so quiet, we are all surprised.

Covered in the white vernix that has kept his skin protected in the amniotic fluid, he quickly turns a bright pink from crying. I whisper to him softly, letting him know everything is fine. He settles at the sound of my voice, and looks suspiciously around him. He has a grumpy little face. He looks so English, like his daddy. Like a grumpy little old Englishman. I ease him back down into the water, and he begins to relax. Nilakantan peers over the edge of the tub at him, smiling at his grumpy countenance. "Well, I guess the next one will be a girl, huh?"

He was right.

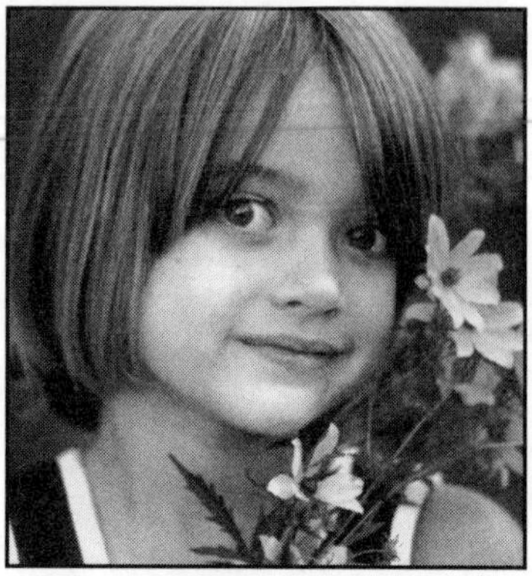

chapter 22

Thanksgiving Surprise

Rani Angela, born November 26, 1993, 1:32 A.M., twenty-two and a half inches long, weighing eight pounds, four ounces.

Three years later, I was waiting again. Our baby was due November 29, 1993. Having had Nataraja eight days late, I figured this baby would be late too. I expected her to come sometime during the first week of December, which is why I was completely surprised by Rani's earlier arrival.

November 25, 1993

Thanksgiving morning and I am once again anxiously awaiting a baby. I'm looking forward to today, to enjoying the company of family and friends, to good food, and fun. Thanksgiving seems particularly appropriate this year, with the evidence of prosperity so obvious in the new baby.

I'm having contractions, as usual. But this morning they're a little different; more crampy and painful. I wonder if this means anything.

Mary told me yesterday that there are more "false" labors after holidays and special events than at any other time of year. The large meals are said to be the blame as they often stimulate contractions. I do not believe it though. I tried the "large meal" technique with Nataraja and it got me nowhere. Still, as the contractions are still coming, I decide to have Mary come over and check my cervix for dilation, just to be sure. Her plans for Thanksgiving mean she will be an hour away. I know I'll feel more comfortable with her going if she finds that nothing much is going on.

On checking me, she finds nothing significant. My cervix has softened and has begun to thin, but labor is likely still a week or two away. It's the news I expected and I don't really mind. I have been so looking forward to Thanksgiving, I am glad I won't be missing it. Mary says she will come by and see me tonight on her way back home and Nilakantan and I wrap up the two boys and head to my parents' house to celebrate.

The day passes pleasantly. Lunch is delicious. I eat as much as I can with the baby so big. Everyone I see asks me when the baby is due. I tell them I've still got a week to go, yet. The contractions are still coming every half-hour or so. I note them, but as they are not truly painful, they do not take my attention away from enjoying the day. I figure I will probably have them on and off now until the baby comes so I had better get used to them.

After lunch, we have tea and pumpkin pie, laughing and visiting, and talking about the year past and the rest still to come. Later the left-overs from lunch make a huge dinner. I lie down after dinner, to rest for a while and to time the contractions that are still coming irregularly. For twenty-five minutes, I have no contractions. I realize the contractions I had were just from the excitement of the day.

It is almost nine o'clock by now. The boys have fallen asleep on the floor. We decide to leave them there. Before we head out, I use the restroom and notice some sticky, pinkish mucus on my underwear. I wonder if that is the mucus plug. I know you can lose the mucus plug days, or even weeks, before beginning labor, but I am excited anyway. I have never lost my mucus plug before. On the way out the door, I tell my mother about it. She smiles at me excitedly and says that maybe this is it. I tell her I don't think so. My contractions have begun again since I got up from resting, but they are still irregular.

At home, I take a nice, long bath. We've put a new tub in the house, and the bath is now deep enough to cover my abdomen. I stay in there a long time. My contractions are still coming. I use them as a practice session; breathing deeply, focusing on relaxing all of my muscles, visualizing my cervix opening. In the tub, I relax from the day.

Once in bed, though, I am unable to sleep. My contractions seem more painful, now, and are coming every seven to ten minutes. At ten thirty, Mary calls. I tell her what is happening and she says she will stop by to see me on her way home in about an hour.

The house is warm with a fire burning in the stove and quiet with the boys gone. I sit in a rocking chair by the fire. Nilakantan sits close by in another chair. We make tea and spend the time waiting for Mary, talking and relaxing.

Mary arrives at 11:25. She sits with me for a few minutes as I have a contraction. It is strong and long enough that she wants to see what is going on with my cervix. On checking me she finds I am six centimeters dilated already. We are all surprised. I didn't even know I was in labor.

Nilakantan and Mary go into high speed, setting up the tub and hose and starting to fill it. I pace across the floor. Now that I have realized I am in labor, the contractions change, becoming stronger, longer, and closer together. Because I didn't know I was in labor, active labor is upon me without my having to wait through the early phase to get to this stage. It makes the labor seem very powerful.

My contractions have jumped from being seven to ten minutes apart to being three to four. Each contraction is powerful, stronger than the last. Even so, I do not find them painful. When each one comes, I remember to relax all my muscles and to focus on allowing my cervix to open.

I know the tub has only just begun to fill and I am longing for the water already. I want to get in now, but I have to wait. When it is only half full, I decide I'm done waiting. They quickly add cold water to bring the temperature down to where it is cool enough, and then I get in. The water is warm and soothing, surrounding me. I relax into it, grateful for the comfort as my contractions continue to come stronger and closer together.

Nilakantan has called my parents to tell them it is time for them to come over; the baby's birth in imminent. He tells them to hurry, but they had been up since six o'clock that morning. They needed coffee before they could make it over. He calls them again, and a third time, telling them if they don't come now, they will miss the baby's birth.

I don't care if they make it or not, and I only barely hear him as he makes the calls. The labor is strong and powerful, each contraction building on the last. Transition comes and goes before I even know it. My parents arrive and I start pushing. Pushing is easy and the baby's head crowns in minutes. Next the shoulders, and then the rest of the baby. Mary feels for the sex—a girl.

Mary brings her up to the surface of the water. She is so pretty—wide-eyed, with dimples. I want to hold her. Mary tries to hand her to me, but Nilakantan still has hold of my arms from supporting me while I pushed her out. I tell him to let go, but he doesn't hear me. He is completely absorbed by his daughter. I can hear him saying, "Oh, my God." I flap my arms, trying to get his attention. I have to tell him three times to let go before he hears me.

I take the baby into my arms and snuggle her close to me. Looking into her eyes, I can see she is one hundred percent there. Where Nataraja had an other-worldly quality to him, this little girl is completely present. So many thoughts run through my head as I look down at her. I know what she may go through as a woman in this world. I know what pain and happiness await her as she grows. My heart already aches in anticipation of the challenges she will face, and warms with the knowledge of the joy she will have. It is such a different feeling from what I felt when the boys were born. I recognize the difference and realize I have become a new mother once again.

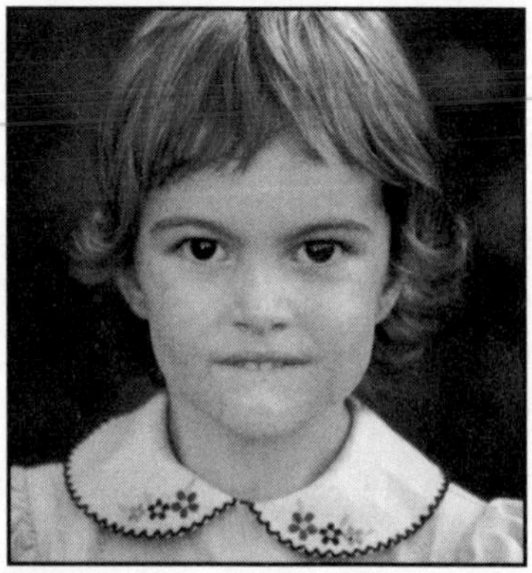

chapter 23

A Hospital Stay, and Then a Home Birth

Madhuri Shana, born June 4, 1996, 6:36 P.M., twenty-two and a half inches long, weighing eight pounds, eleven ounces.

Rani's birth was so quick and easy, we almost didn't have time to fill the tub. After such an easy third birth, I figured my fourth would be even easier, and I worried that we wouldn't have time to fill the tub. Madhuri's birth proved that no matter how many times it happens, birth is never predictable.

Madhuri's birth was preceded by so many stressful occurrences that by the time her due date arrived, I was actually relieved that she hadn't been born. Because of this, I experienced none of the anxious waiting that I had with the two boys, neither had I the element of surprise as with Rani's birth. Madhuri waited until exactly the right time, and then she was born.

June 4, 1996:

This morning I wake up grateful that Rani slept through the night for the first time in five days. Before that, it was Nilakantan I was worried about.

On May 9th, three weeks ago, Nilakantan woke up in the middle of the night with violent stomach cramps. He was so sick, he had to be taken to the ER. He spent an entire day there while they treated him for severe dehydration, and then sent him home that evening, uncured, with the probable diagnosis of "stomach flu."

Over the next few days, he seemed to get only marginally better. He could eat very little, was tired all of the time, and five days later, the violent pain began to come back. We returned to the ER. After running more tests, a CT scan showed that he was suffering from a ruptured appendix, and that it had ruptured prior to his first trip to the hospital. Somehow they had missed it.

That night he had emergency surgery.

Fortunately I wasn't aware of the seriousness of his condition as I sat alone in the surgical waiting room while they operated. It was only later that I realized how lucky he was to be alive.

The operation took two and a half hours. He came through it well, but was very sick and had to remain in the hospital for a week while they gave him intravenous antibiotics to kill the infection caused by the rupture. For the first four days I stayed with him, sleeping on a cot at the bottom of his bed, all of our children staying with my parents.

On the morning of the fourth day, I began having regular contractions accompanied by extreme agitation. It seemed that the stress was catching up with me and we determined that I would stay at home for the rest of his hospital stay, only coming in during the day to visit.

We told the surgeons who were caring for Nilakantan that I needed to go home in case the baby came. After all, I didn't want to give birth in the hospital! We told them should I go into labor, we would need an ambulance to rush me home. They found it extremely funny as the maternity ward was on the floor above us.

Nilakantan remained in the hospital for seven days. After that, they let him come home on the condition that I would change the dressing on his incision site three times a day. It was very difficult once he got home and the reality of his condition, and thus our situation, hit us. Our baby was due in two weeks, Nilakantan was unable to walk well, to drive for six weeks, or to lift anything over ten pounds. As big as a barrel by now, I wasn't much better.

It occurred to me at that time that there must be a higher power because I would never plan my life that way. It was like some big cosmic joke. One that we would, hopefully, find funny one day.

As it was, Nilakantan's parents came from England to lend a hand. Between their help, and that of my parents, all our bases were covered.

And so, we all sit and wait for the new arrival. Doris and Don, Nilakantan's parents, have been here a week now, but the baby has not made an appearance. I did have one good "false" labor, complete with the tub filled, and the video camera set up (we've decided to film this birth) but the baby didn't come.

Yesterday, Mary said the baby was still high and it seems like it will be another week. We're all a little saddened by this. If the baby waits that long, Doris and Don won't get to see the baby before they go back to England. But it's good they're here, anyway, as I don't know how we'd manage without them.

Rani smiles at me this morning looking more herself after a good night's sleep. I notice her lower left jaw appears swollen. For the last five days, she hasn't been sleeping well, and has been crying so much; I know she's been in pain. We suspected her teeth were causing the problem, and took her to the dentist yesterday to get them checked, but she wouldn't even open her mouth so her teeth could be looked at. Now, I wonder from the swelling if she has an abscessed tooth.

I gingerly put my finger into her mouth and feel a large lump on her gums, below her molars. Just as I touch it, it pops. I am relieved to find it, now having a reason for her suffering. I stand up off the bed to get the pain medication from atop the bookshelf and as I sit back down, I feel a little pop inside of me and liquid begins to trickle out, feeling warm like pee. I realize my water bag must have broken.

I give Rani her medicine and stand up off the bed. As I go through the kitchen on the way to the bathroom, I meet Doris in the hallway. I say, "Rani has an abscessed tooth and my waterbag has just broken." She's not sure whether to be happy about the baby coming or sad for Rani. "Right," she says, and we both laugh.

While Doris and Don help out getting the boys ready for school, I call the dentist to get a prescription of antibiotics for Rani, then I call Mary to let her know my water broke. I've placed a cloth in my underwear to catch the water and it feels very strange. Every time I get up from sitting or stand up from bending over, a gush of fluid runs out. I decide to wait for Mary sitting down. We put a plastic drop cloth over the couch and cover it with a towel and I sit down.

Doris and Don leave to take the boys to school and then go to get Rani's prescription, which leaves Nilakantan and me alone. He is doing much better after a week at home and gets me glasses of water and tea while we wait for Mary. It's a beautiful day, with the temperature only in the mid-eighties, cooler than usual for this time of year.

Mary comes at nine o'clock. I'm not having many contractions yet, and the ones I have had weren't painful. I don't think I've dilated any yet, and because there is a risk of infection now that the water bag has broken, Mary decides not to check yet.

Every once in a while I get a contraction. Short and not very long at the peak, I know they will have to get much stronger for the baby to be born. I remember the power of Rani's birth, and I think it will probably still be a while before this baby is born.

Our photographer, Chandra Schoonover, has arrived, along with Mary. As well as being a dear friend, Chandra is also a masseuse and she spends some time on each of us, massaging the tension from our necks and shoulders.

By eleven o'clock, not much has changed. Mary decides to check me, though we both think my cervix will not be much dilated due to the lightness and infrequency of the contractions. It turns out I am four centimeters already and it looks as if the baby may come soon.

Mary fills the tub, with Chandra's help this time, as Nilakantan is still unable to do much. My parents are called and informed of my progress. They decide to wait out most of the labor at their house where Doris and Don are also waiting.

Once it's full, I don't feel like getting in the tub. My labor is still too slow for me to want to get into the water. I wander around waiting for things to pick up. My contractions are coming irregularly, ten to twenty minutes apart and still short at the peak. I try walking outside to help to get the labor going, but it's hot, so I come back inside. I eat a light meal and then rest.

At two-thirty Mary checks my cervix again. I am making progress, but the baby is still high and needs to come down quite a bit. We decide to empty the tub as it is getting cold and I still have no inclination to get in.

I am restless and go outside onto our back deck. A storm is rolling in on dark clouds. I have read that the energy generated by a storm can stimulate labor. I wonder if this one will help mine. While I am walking, Mary suggests I try rolling my nipples between my fingers to see if that will help to stimulate contractions. When nipples are stimulated a natural hormone called oxytocin is released causing the uterus to contract which can help with a slow labor.

It seems to help and as the storm breaks in earnest, I ask for the tub to be filled. At four thirty it is ready and I get in. The contractions are stronger and painful enough that I am grateful when the tub is ready. They are still short at the peak, though, and five or six minutes apart.

In the tub, I relax completely. This is so familiar and comforting. I laugh and joke in between contractions, and breathe through each one. My labor continues in the same odd pattern that it has shown all along, with contractions coming at irregular intervals and being short at the peak. Even though this is the case, my labor becomes increasingly painful, more so than I remember from my other births. Each contraction seems to roll right through me, leaving me exhausted.

Mary wants to check the baby's heartbeat. I get out of the tub. Half an hour ago, I was laughing and joking, now I barely hear what people are saying to me. The baby's heartbeat sounds good and I am nine centimeters dilated, but the baby still has not dropped down into the birth canal. Nine centimeters, I know, could mean a half an hour of labor yet to go. I feel so discouraged, the contractions are so painful, I want the labor to be over.

I get back in the tub and another contraction hits me. It goes and minutes later another one comes. As the peak of this one slides away, I suddenly have an overwhelming urge to push. I push with all my might and I feel the baby moving down through my pelvic bones to the vaginal opening where her head crowns. Mary tells me to slow down, there's no need to hurry. She says to pant like I did with Nataraja, and the baby's head eases out. I reach down and rub the baby's head, welcoming, marveling. On that one push, she is almost born.

For ninety seconds, I wait for another contraction to push her out the rest of the way. Mary's hands are on the baby's head along with mine. She says she can feel the umbilical cord is wrapped twice around the baby's neck, and that it is still pulsing; a sign that the baby is receiving blood and oxygen through the cord.

Even though I have no contraction, Mary tells me to push. As I push, the shoulders are born, one first, then the other, followed by the rest of the baby. While Mary is busy under the water sliding the umbilical cord over the baby's head to unwrap it from the neck, I am checking for the sex and finding I have another girl. I am so happy. Secretly, I wanted another girl.

The cord unwraps a total of three and a half times. Then Mary brings the baby up out of the water and lays her in my arms. She is quiet and still. Outside, the storm has gone and the sun breaking through the clouds streams in through the kitchen window and casts a soft light on her. Mary rubs her back and massages her stomach trying to stimulate her to breathe. She coughs a little and sputters, then is quiet again. Finally, Mary flicks the bottom of her feet and immediately she cries heartbreaking wails. Not the grumpy, angry wails of Nataraja, hers are the sad sort of crying that tugs at your heart. I lean over and whisper to her, comforting. After a moment she quiets. Her eyes gazing up at me look far away and otherwordly and deep like the bottom of the sea.

She has clasped the medallion I always wear in her fist and doesn't let it go even as I lean over and ease her body back down into the water. Nilakantan leans in to look at her, holding a hand up to shield her from the late afternoon sun. We are both so happy to see her, having so recently been reminded of the preciousness and fragility of life. She seems an even greater gift for the reminder.

Madhuri's birth was the most difficult of all my experiences. Having the umbilical cord wrapped so many times around her neck is probably what prevented her from moving down into the birth canal until the very end, when I pushed her all the way to crowning on the one push. And her remaining high in the birth canal is what caused the contractions to be so painful for me.

Once Madhuri's head was born, the ninety seconds that went by while we waited for another contraction caused some pressure to be built up in her head. This caused the whites of her eyes to be filled with blood, and her cheeks and chin to sustain purple bruises. In addition to this, her collarbone was broken. A relatively common occurrence called a "spring break"—I sustained one during my own birth—Madhuri's was probably caused by her very rapid descent down the birth canal.

In reviewing this experience later, I had to ask myself if I felt she would have been better off in a hospital setting. I realized we were very fortunate that Madhuri sustained no lasting damage from the umbilical cord being wrapped around her neck, and from moving down the birth canal so quickly.

From what I have learned of hospital practice, though, I have become certain she had a better chance at home. My labor could have been considered "dysfunctional" in the hospital setting due to the contractions being light, irregular, and short through the peak. From this determination, pitocin, a drug given to stimulate uterine contractions, may have been administered. I am not sure Madhuri would have survived the longer, harder, and more frequent contractions caused by the pitocin. From this drug, her blood supply, which naturally decreases during each contraction, as noted by a decreased heart rate, may have become too low to sustain her.

There is no way for me to know if this would have been the case. It is just a feeling I have, a sense of knowing that the choice I made was right. Knowing what could have happened to her, I find myself grateful everyday that she was born safe and sound.

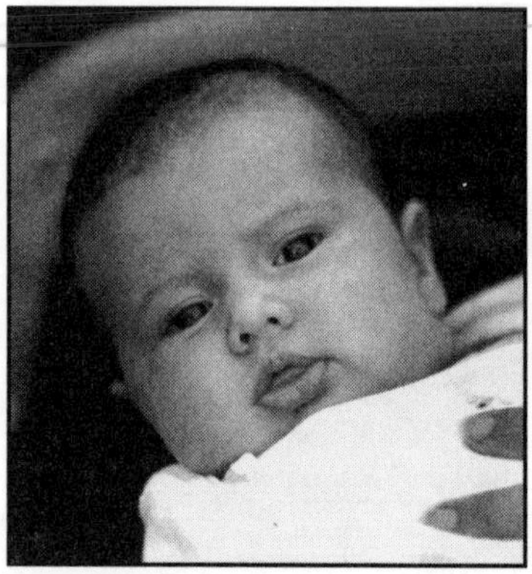

chapter 24

Birth Center Waterbirth

Lalita Karensa, born July 27, 1999, 11:36 A.M., twenty-two inches long, eight pounds, eleven ounces.

There is nothing quite like waiting for a baby to be born. Your whole life goes on hold while you count and time contractions, you fold and re-fold baby clothes, and you wake up every morning wondering if today will be the day. This experience of endless waiting is universally prevalent and frustrating. So much so that by the time your due date arrives, and often goes by without the birth of your baby, you begin to feel you would do anything to have your baby be born.

I think this may be a part of the reason why so many women are willing to have their labors induced. Particularly when you couple this endless waiting with two or three trips to the doctor only to be sent home because the labor was "false." Women can get pretty worn down by this. They can lose their courage, their confidence, and their belief in their own ability. No one likes to arrive at the doctor's feeling ill, only to be sent home without a diagnosis. Laboring women experience this type of thing all of the time.

This is another reason why I knew I wanted to give birth at home. I couldn't imagine having to leave my home and travel somewhere in order to give birth. It seemed so disruptive, so wrong. I wondered how I would be able to relax and focus inward while in transit, and even more, in the unfamiliar surroundings of a hospital, with people I didn't know surrounding me, with bright lights glaring.

Fortunately, I have been lucky enough not to have to have that experience of birth. But I did give birth to one of my babies out of my home. Lalita Karensa, my fifth baby: born in water, just not born at home.

It gave me a lot of understanding to have had to leave my home to birth Lalita. I suddenly understood a woman's inability to relax and let her labor happen in the hospital setting. Nothing about the idea of having to leave my home was comforting or reassuring. All I wanted to do in labor was hunker down and have my baby. The thought of having to travel while in labor made me feel very tense and uncertain. So much so that I made three trips to the birth center, prior to the baby actually being born.

At the Birth Center of the Blue Ridge in Charlottesville, Virginia, my surroundings were far better than they would have been in the hospital. The rooms were designed to mimic the home environment, with a double bed, a couch, and a few comfortable chairs in each room, along with the jacuzzi "birthing" tub. There was a kitchenette down the hall for food items, and a waiting room with a couch and a TV and VCR for loved ones not in the birthing room.

Nilakantan, the children, my parents, and other family and friends, were all welcome to be present for the birth, as per my wishes. The midwives were supportive and encouraging, and willingly allowed me to labor at my own speed. Which was just as well as I spent an entire night there waiting to feel comfortable enough in the unfamiliar surroundings to be able to relax fully and let my baby be born.

July 26, 1999:

Today has been almost exactly the same as every other day for the last three weeks. I wake early to contractions that slow down once I get up and pick back up again in the afternoon. Today, however, my contractions are accompanied by a bloody show, the presence of which could signify that my cervix has begun to dilate.

I am hesitant to believe it, even though my contractions are coming every eight to ten minutes. In the last three weeks I have gone to the birth center three times, only to be told not much was happening. The last time I went, they told me I was three centimeters dilated and over fifty percent effaced, but was not yet in labor.

The baby is in a good position, and is very low. Already this birth differs from Madhuri's. My fear now is of not knowing in time. The birth center is over forty-five miles away. Too far to travel if this baby decides to make a hasty entry. This thought is constantly in my mind as I go through each day counting contractions. When Madhuri was born, my labor did not get hard until the last two hours. I remember this now. I do not want to be driving for an hour in the car while I am in hard labor. Thus, every "set" of regular contractions has me ready for flight to the birth center.

I realize I am not feeling relaxed about this birth at all.

On the phone this morning, my sister Cassi, who had her first baby in water and her second baby in the hospital without water, told me the next time I had regular contractions, I needed to go to the birth center and get really settled in, and to tell myself I was not leaving until I had my baby, no matter if it took three days.

I think about that. I'm having regular contractions now. But I've had them for days, how can I know this is it? I look at the clock: three P.M. I decide to rest for an hour and then see if I am feeling any differently. I lie down but can't rest because the contractions are more painful when I lie down.

I get up and sit in the rocking chair instead. All the kids have gone to play at my sister's house and it is so quiet and still, so peaceful. I have a cup of tea, and the contractions are still coming.

When I use the bathroom, I notice more bloody show. I know this could be a sign of labor starting. I decide to go to the birth center.

At four o'clock my mother and I leave after having called Nilakantan to let him know what is happening. He is still at work but plans to meet us at the center later. I kiss the kids goodbye and tell them our baby might be coming. Originally I had wanted the kids to be at the birth center when the baby was born, knowing how important early bonding can be for the children and the new baby. But I can't bring myself to drag them into the center for a fourth time in three weeks. And I don't know how long I will be there. I decide they are better off at my sister's house.

The drive is pleasant. It is hot outside, with the temperature in the nineties, as is usual for July in central Virginia, and we run the air conditioning to stay cool. My mother laughs and talks with me as we drive in. I have been feeling very anxious since we left and I notice by the time we arrive in Charlottesville, where the birthing center is located, my contractions have slowed down. This makes me feel even more anxious and I take a few deep breaths to relax.

Jackie and Sandy, the midwife team, meet us at the center. We have decided to have photographs of this birth taken and

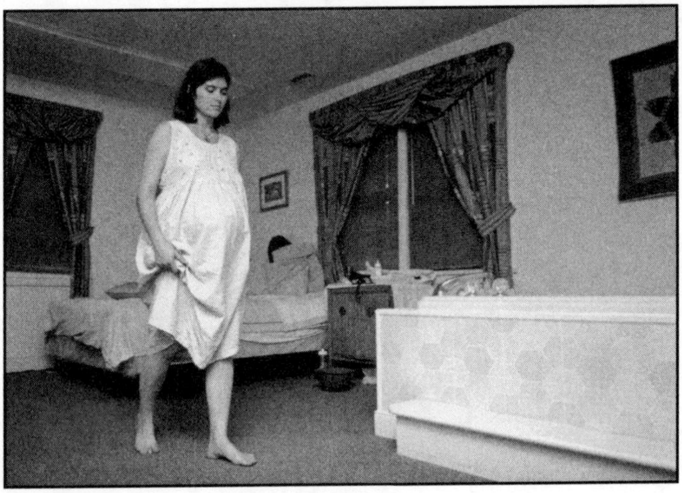

Stephanie Gross, our photographer, is there as well. They are all smiles and welcoming, joking with me and reassuring me. The center had eight women due between mid-July and mid-August. All the other women have delivered. Only I

am left. They tell me no one else is due for another three weeks which means I can stay there as long as I need to in order to birth my baby. I appreciate their offer of accommodation; it makes me feel more at home.

In the room I will be birthing in, I spend time by myself, trying to get used to the feel of the place. I like it here, the rooms are inviting and pleasant and the jacuzzi tub in the corner is reassuring. Nilakantan and my father have arrived and I can hear everyone in the other room laughing and talking. I wander in to see them and everyone asks me how I am doing. I tell them not much different, and then I sit in a rocking chair and listen to them talk for a while. It's a neat feeling, now that I'm here. It feels more like a slumber party than a birth.

The evening is spent with me alternating walking and sitting in the chair, but my labor has not picked up. Finally, I'm tired and want to go to bed. Jackie checks my cervix for dilation before I go to lie down. I'm nervous as she does, knowing this check will tell whether or not I am in labor.

I am four centimeters dilated and officially in labor. She says the baby is good and low, she can feel the head. And she tells me, judging from the circumference of the head that she can feel, this baby is going to be smaller than the others, between seven and a half and eight pounds. A smaller baby sounds good to me.

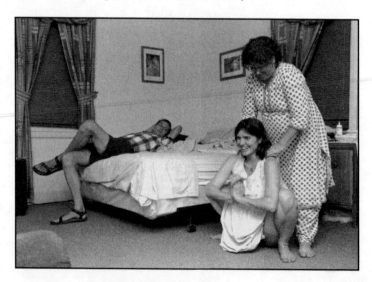

Because active labor has not begun yet, we all decide to rest. In the birthing room, Nilakantan and I take the bed, Mother takes some pillows and sleeps on the floor at the foot of the bed, and Dad takes the couch. Stephanie is on a couch in another room, and Jackie and Sandy are downstairs in the basement rooms.

Everyone settles in to sleep. My contractions are too painful to sleep lying down, so I prop myself up with pillows and drift away. I have not been hungry since this afternoon, but I make sure to drink a carbohydrate drink, rich in minerals and electrolytes, to keep my strength up. Through the night, I drift in and out of sleep and make countless trips to the bathroom to pee. The contractions continue all night long, sometimes getting stronger and more regular, and then tapering off again.

At six A.M., I shake off the last vestiges of sleep, stretch and get up. Nilakantan and Mom and Dad awake with me. "Where's that baby?" my Dad asks. I just smile and shrug. "On the way, I hope."

Coffee is put on and doughnuts are sent for. The birthing team is hungry. I find out my baby sister, Poorna, has spent the night outside sleeping in her car with two of her friends, holding vigil. I am so touched by this. She is the doughnut runner, sent back out again just as she returns to get more coffee.

Mom and I are alone together in the birthing room. Nilakantan is looking in a baby name book, and Dad has left for a meeting with clients. Mother tells me he is worried about missing the birth, and is going to be as quick as he can.

I'm tired from so many contractions and from only getting a little sleep and my contractions are becoming more painful. Mom asks me if I want the tub filled. I don't believe I am in active labor, but I decide to have it filled anyway, as I know it will be relaxing to be in the water.

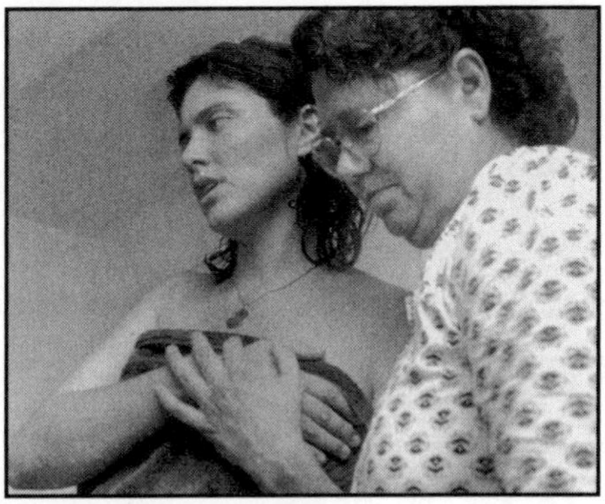

By nine forty-five the tub is ready. I feel slightly spoiled looking into the beautiful jacuzzi tub. A far cry from the horse trough I birthed the other babies in. But once I get in, I realize the water feels just the same. I'm so tired, I need very little coaxing to relax deeply. I relax so much that my labor slows down. My mother notices this, and tells me I have to get out and walk. I listen to her because she is my mother. I'm supposed to listen to her. She helps me out of the tub and we walk back and forth around the room.

My labor has been long. I have been at the center for fifteen hours already, but it has not been hard. The contractions are not really painful, they are just there, erratically coming and going. When I start to feel too much discomfort, I get back in the water and when my labor slows down, at my mother's urging, I get back out to walk.

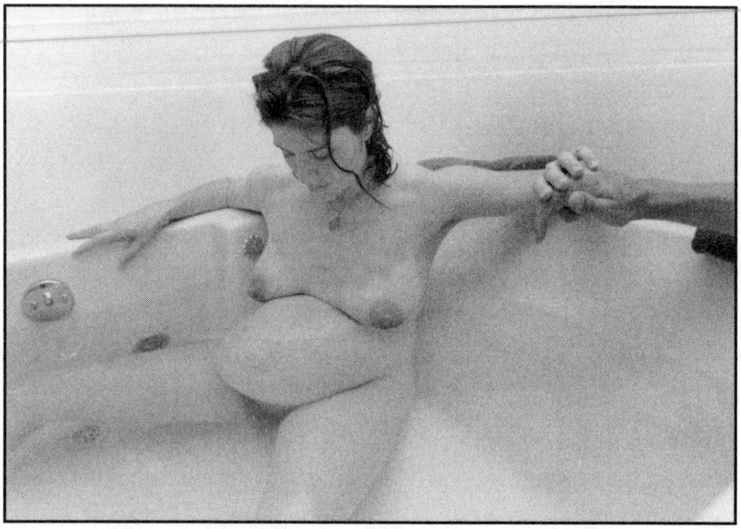

After a while, though, I am too tired and decide I want to sleep. It's close to eleven o'clock by now. Mom thinks resting is a bad idea and suggests Jackie check my cervix for progress before I rest. If I am a good way along, Mother tells me I ought to go ahead and have the baby and rest later. She asks me what I think. Right now I think my mother is pushy, but she's probably right.

On examining me Jackie finds that I am over six centimeters dilated. I am so glad to hear it and for the first time I accept that I am actually in labor. She also says that my cervix is very soft and stretchy. She is able to stretch it to eight centimeters while she is examining me. She says the baby is ready to come and all it will take to dilate the last two centimeters is for me to exert a little pressure on my cervix from inside by squatting.

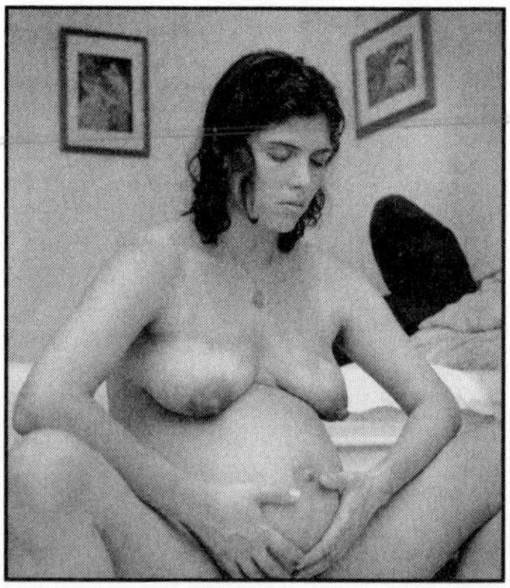

I squat outside of the tub during my contractions. Consciously I focus on my cervix opening, and on moving the baby down. I can feel the baby begin to shift lower. And my contractions begin to feel a little like pushing. I look at Jackie surprised. It has only been a few minutes, yet I know I am nearly there. She asks me if I want to get back in the water to have the baby. I nod and Mother helps me to climb back in.

I tell her to go get Nilakantan and Dad. They come in and I am in transition already. Nilakantan comes behind me, to sit at my back and lend support. As the contractions are coming hard now, I am glad he is there. I feel myself drawing in, bringing all of my attention inside, to work through this pain. As each contraction comes, I know I am one step closer to the birth of the baby. I note this fact at the beginning and end of each contraction. I know I am close, and recognize a shift in the energy of this contraction, at the same time.

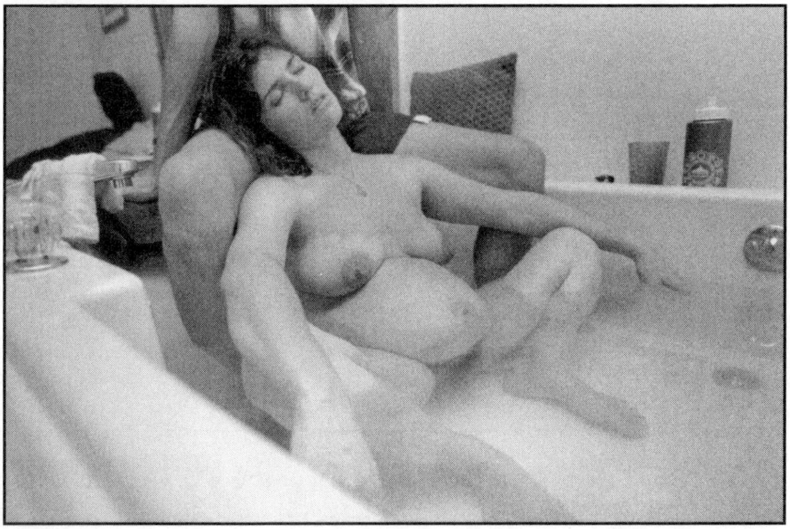

Jackie reaches inside me and pushes back a last edge of the cervix that was still in the way, then tells me to push. The contraction is really painful, and as I push, I feel the baby move past the cervix and feel the pressure as the baby moves down through the birth canal. There is intense burning as the head crowns, and then comes out. Jackie has her hands

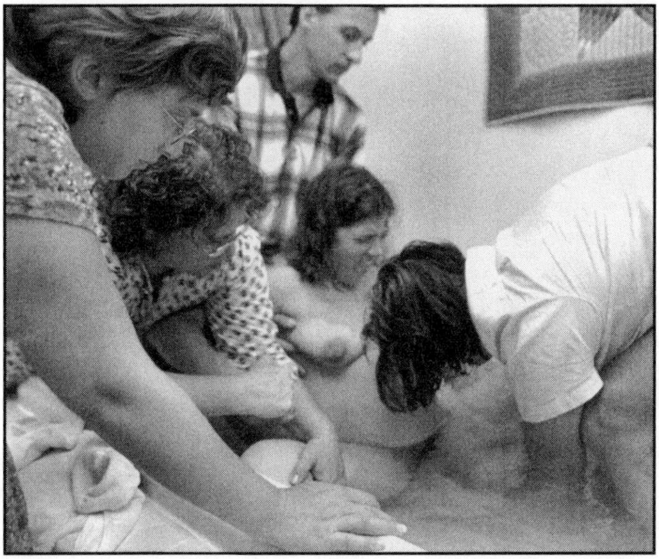

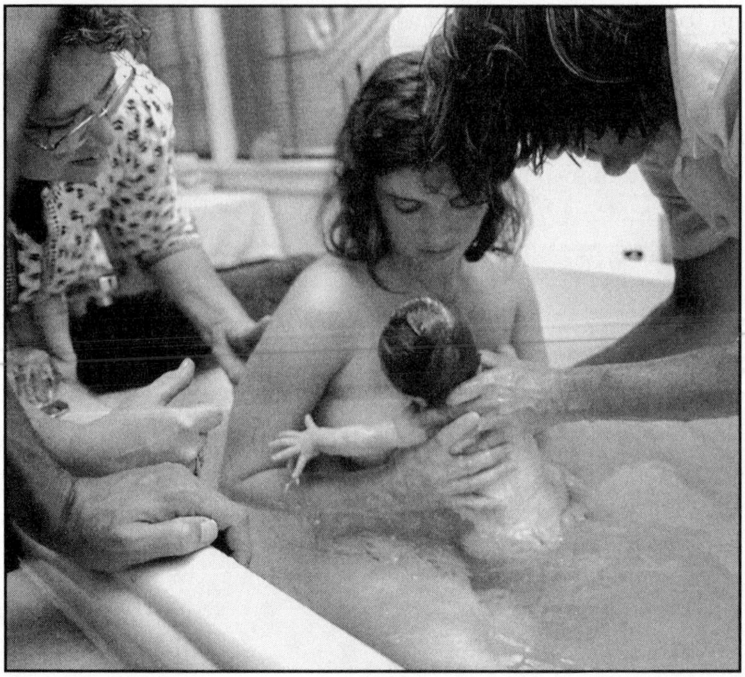

on the baby's head and says, "That's a much bigger head than I thought it was." Behind me Nilakantan laughs and says, "Tell us something we didn't know. Our babies have always been bigger than people have guessed."

I can feel Jackie pulling gently on the baby's head, trying to coax her out. She says the baby's shoulders feel stuck. She tries for a minute more to shift the shoulders, while I remain squatting and then she asks me to flip over so I am leaning on my arms on the edge of the tub and my belly is facing down. In this position, the baby comes out easily with another push, swishing into the water. I can't see anything from this position, so I sit back immediately, looking for the baby

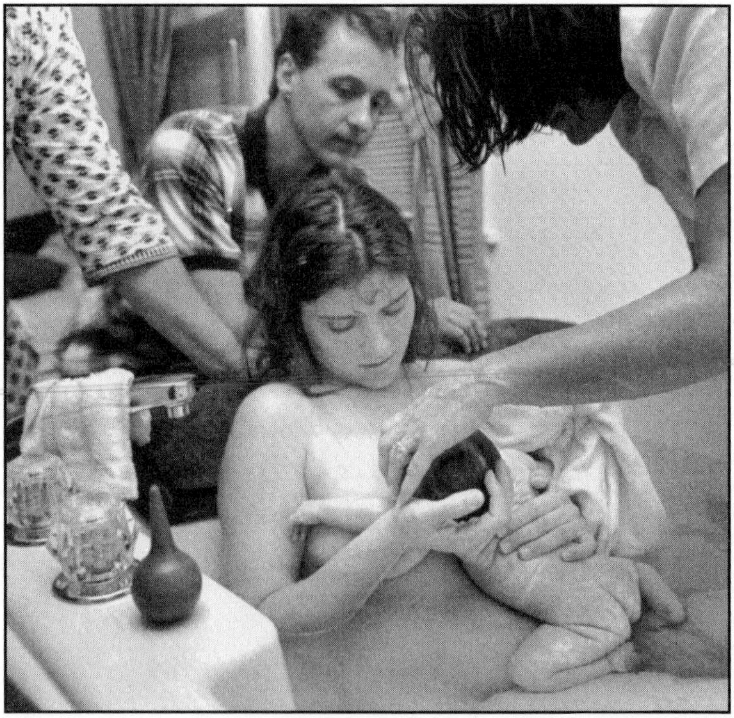

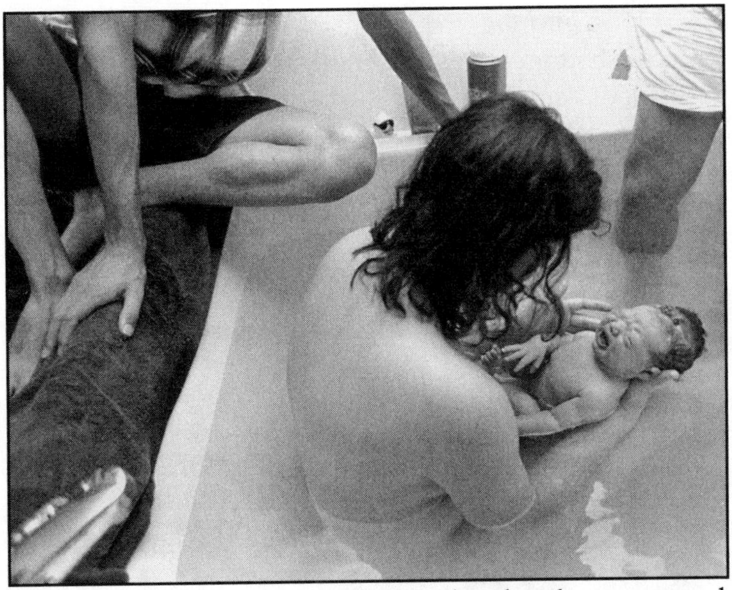

who is still under the water. I can't find her because she is under my leg.

Jackie has hold of her and she brings her up to the surface, handing her to me and telling me we have another girl. I look into the baby's far-away eyes. She is not breathing and I speak to her, feeling as if I am calling to her soul. I ask her if she has plans to breathe sometime today, and I tell her that air is necessary. I can see she isn't here yet. Jackie is working on her, rubbing her back and her belly. The cord is still pulsing, so she is in no danger. But Jackie and I decide at the same moment that the time has come for her to breathe.

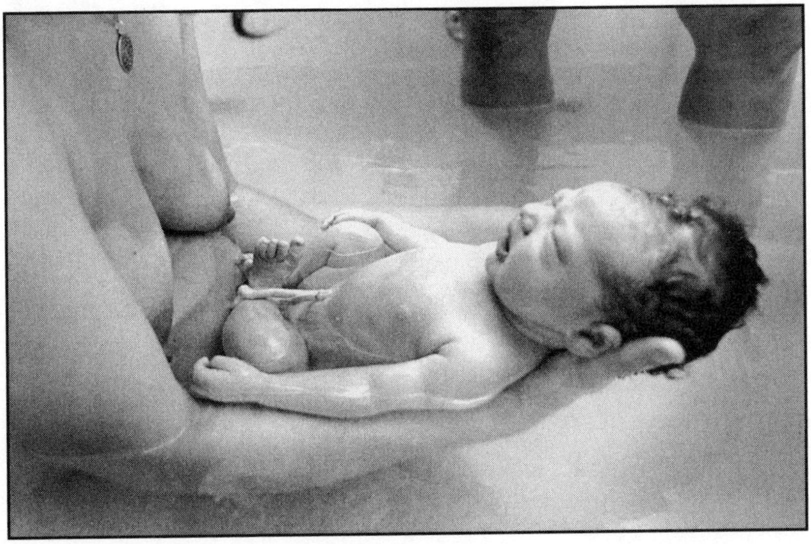

I hold her head and look into her eyes and tell her to breathe and Jackie flicks the bottom of her feet. Startled into breathing, she cries. She looks so upset. Her bottom lip is stuck out as she wails. Her cries sound offended, as if she can't believe we would do something so cruel as to flick her

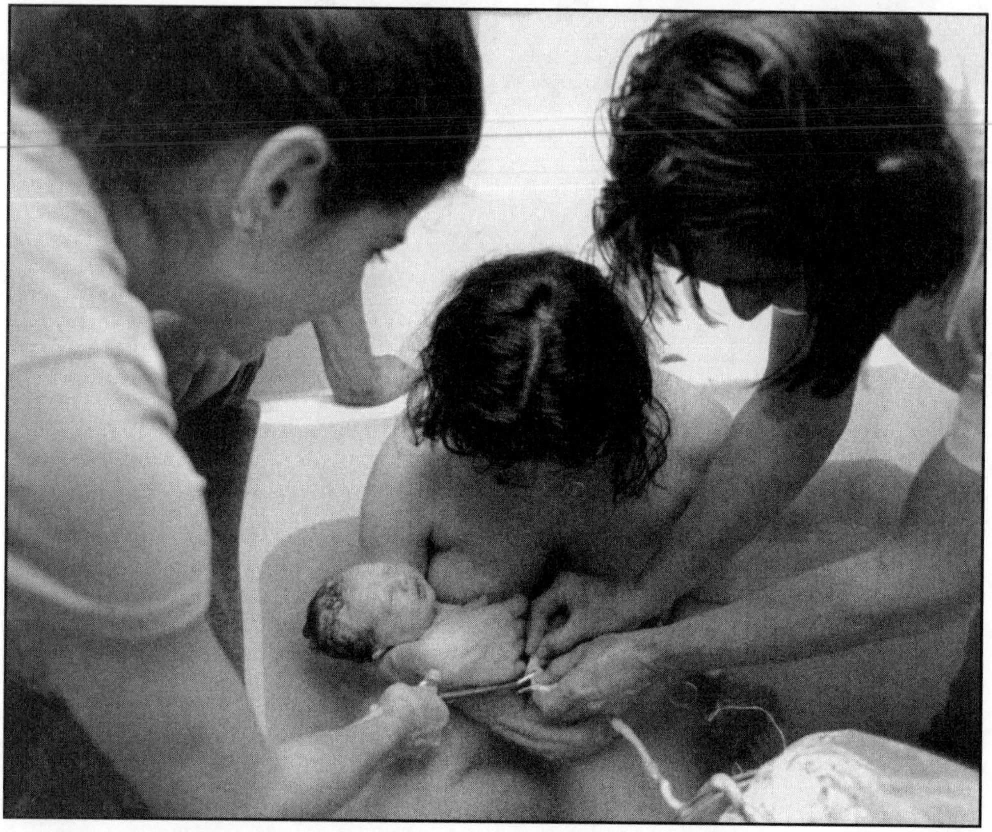

feet. I talk to her soothingly and laugh, and all the seven people gathered close around the tub to witness her birth, laugh with me.

I notice now that Poorna is here. She arrived back here with the coffee, just as the baby was being born. I'm glad she was here to witness the birth, and that her all-night vigil was rewarded with being there for the birth. She looks awed by what she saw, and when she is asked if she would like to cut the umbilical cord, she does not hesitate to be a part of this birth experience. Poorna is the last of my parents' six

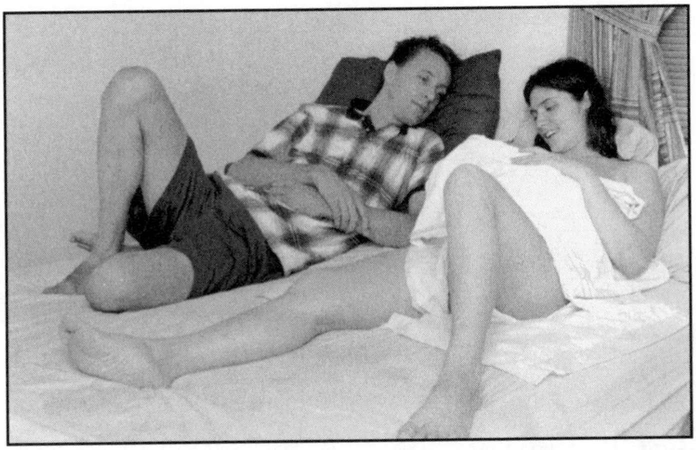

children. I wonder if this will turn out to be my last birth. If so, I am glad she was there to witness it.

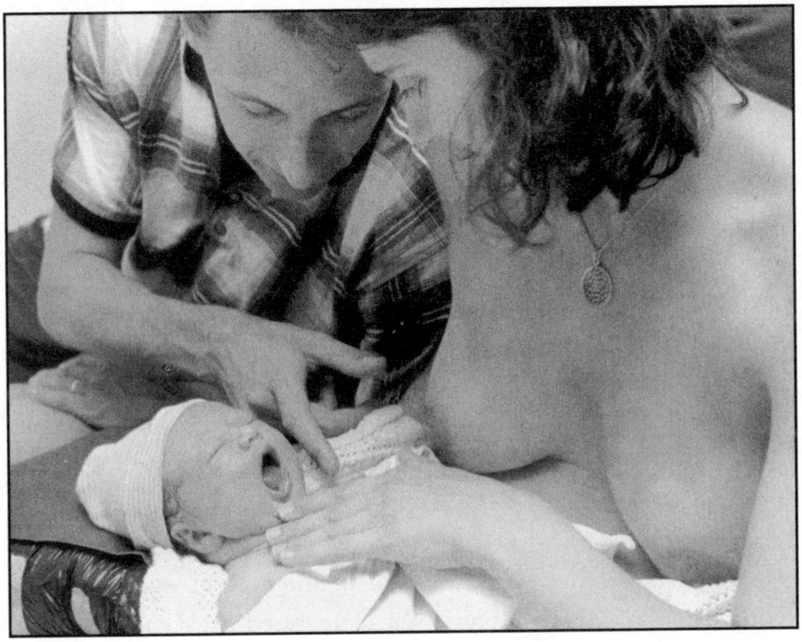

chapter 25

My Sister's Waterbirth

Thurston Lewis Stish, born September 8, 1996, twenty-two and a half inches long, weighing nine pounds, four ounces.

This was the first time I had been at a birth where I was not the one having the baby. It is a very different experience, watching a woman in labor. My sister showed strength and courage. I have never seen anything as amazing as she was while she pushed her baby out.

My eldest sister Cassi became pregnant at thirty-three with her first baby when I was pregnant with my fourth. She had been trying to get pregnant for about a year, so it was with great joy that she took the news that she was pregnant at last.

While thoroughly excited about the baby, Cassi was very fearful of the actual birth. Completely against the Western medical system, she was determined to have a natural, home birth, but for one who is admittedly a "total wimp" when it comes to pain, she wondered how she would ever make it through labor and delivery without needing drugs for the pain. Waterbirth for her was like finding a candle in a cavern; it gave her something real and solid that would help guide her through an unknown experience.

Mary was to be her midwife, as well, and her husband, George, our parents, and I were to be present as her support team. When Cassi first asked me to attend her birth, I had reservations. I had just had Madhuri, and her birth had been challenging and more painful than the three before her. I wasn't sure I wanted to be at another birth that would certainly remind me of my own that had been only a few months earlier. But it was very important to Cassi that I be there. She said I was her living, breathing example that labor could be gone through and survived, so having me about would remind her of that.

September 6, 1996:

Today dawned windy and gray as Hurricane Fran beat down on us for the second day in a row. Mother called me this morning, letting me know that Cassi was having contractions that were coming pretty regularly. With the weather we've been having I am not surprised. An everyday thunderstorm can cause a woman to go into labor, never mind a hurricane. And even though it is still two weeks until her due date, Cassi has already lost her mucus plug and the wagers have begun on how long she will hold out before the baby is born. The day passes, and though Cassi is tired and cranky, she is not yet in labor.

September 7:

Over breakfast this morning, we lost electricity. Though not an unusual occurence in rural Virginia, the loss of the electricity this morning is significant. Cassi has planned for a home waterbirth, so if the electricity does not come back on in time, I wonder what will happen.

At my mother's house, I see Cassi, who is making breakfast when I walk in. She seems a little tired and much distressed. Her contractions have begun again, and though the rain is still pouring down, the temperature has begun to rise. With no water available for showers, and no air conditioning, she is facing a day of heat and humidity with no way to alleviate the discomfort. She and George decide to go to a motel in a town twenty miles away to shower, rest, and regroup.

Mid-afternoon, the contractions are back, much stronger and more painful. Cassi calls Mary to let her know what is happening and she tells them to come home and she will meet them there. At home Cassi calls the electric company. The service man, upon hearing her predicament, tells her the electricity will not be restored to their grid for at least two days. He recommends they evacuate.

I arrive at the house just after Mary does. My Dad comes and lets Cassi know a neighbor has a generator and can draw hot water. Does she still want to try for a waterbirth? She says yes and George and Nilakantan accompany him to help haul water.

Cassi goes into the house and lies down. She finally takes stock of her situation. She has no water for the birthing tub, no fan or air conditioning to keep her cool, no running water for showers or cooking, no CD player for her carefully chosen music. Everything she had dreamed of and planned to help to bring her baby into the world was gone, stripped away by the hurricane. As she thinks of these things, and feels her carefully laid plans unraveling, she realizes there is only one thing she can do to make her situation better and that is to let go. So she counts off each transgression, ticks them off in her head, and mentally allows each one to be let go. "Thy will be done," is her mantra of the moment and her reward is a deep pervading peace settling over her.

At this exact moment, the electricity comes back on.

Relief washes over us all. The world makes sense again.

Mary checks Cassi and she is only one and a half centimeters dilated. Mary can't be sure if it is labor yet; the next few hours will tell. If her cervix dilates any more over the next two hours, then she is in labor. Walking is good if you're trying to decide if labor is here or not. If it is true labor, you will dilate faster; if false, it will usually slow or stop altogether.

Cassi's contractions continue to come and by 4:30, two hours later, she is four and a half centimeters dilated and is declared officially in labor.

The tub is filled and Cassi gets in. She remarked later: "I still remember the feeling of comfort and safety in the water; caressed by Mother Ocean, I never wanted to get out."

Cassi labors in the water and out, working hard to produce her baby. She is not "wimpy" at all. That person has gone and has been replaced by this woman who is becoming a mother. A trial by fire, this journey is not an easy one, but

Cassi is amazing. She sways and rocks back and forth, both in the water and out on all fours. She makes loud, low noises, deep belly sounds that help her to stay focused. Her music plays, soothing her, sage burns in a clam shell and candles cast a soft glow. George gives support, massaging and holding her. My mother and father, Mary, and I wait quietly as Cassi does all the work.

By the time dawn comes, she is pushing with all of her might. A half an hour ago she was listless in between contractions and introverted during them. Now she is vibrant and dynamic with each powerful push. Slowly, the head appears a little at a time. More pushing and all at once he is born. She looks at him as he is laid in her arms and says, "Boy, did you cause me some trouble." We all laugh because we know this is only the beginning.

Cassi's second baby, Charles Tasso Stish (born January 23, 1999), was not able to be born in water. Cassi and George had moved to Pennsylvania, where there was no one in the area who practiced waterbirths. She considered coming down here to stay for the last month until her baby was born, but that would mean George would not be able to be present at the birth. Her only option in Pennsylvania was to depend on the Western medical hospital that she was so opposed to.

She found a group of doctors who were highly recommended. On her first visit, she explained about her first birth, and she told them if she gave birth in their center, she would have certain expectations that they would need to agree upon meeting before she had her baby there. She gave them a written list of her criteria. The hospital board met to see if they could uphold her desires. The answer was yes and from that careful planning, Cassi's second baby was born after only four hours of active labor, making his appearance halfway through James Taylor's "Sweet Baby James."

Cassi felt very positively about this second, very different birth experience. In lieu of the birthing tub, she said she felt the water became a state of mind for her. She did not fear this birth at all. Her only concerns were with where and how she would give birth. Once those things were taken care of to her satisfaction, the rest of her experience was as good as she had hoped. She feels this was solely due to the amazing experience she had had the first time around. It taught her that she wasn't a "total wimp" after all.

Part IV

The Celebration and Afterwards

chapter 26

Congratulations and Welcome

Having just given birth to a new being, the first thing you deserve is a wholehearted congratulations. Congratulations and welcome to the frustrating, wonderful, miraculous, impossible, thoroughly demanding and absolutely fulfilling world of motherhood. Your job is like no other. You are to be on call twenty-four hours a day; you are to give of yourself fully; you are to forget about achieving any personal goals for the time being; you are not to be allowed to shower in peace; and you are to experience a sense of love, devotion and wholehearted commitment unlike anything you have ever known before. With this new person to take care of, your time is no longer your own. Your time, and a large portion of your heart and brain, belong to the baby you hold in your arms.

When we talk about the "miracle of creation," we refer to this: the magic, the miracle of one person in his/her sweetness and innocence transforming the life of another. This miraculous event makes us into mothers. You will be changed by your baby. Expect to be.

And expect to be occasionally resentful of it; expect to miss the good old days when you could pee in peace, eat a meal from beginning to end without twenty-two interruptions, and sleep the night through.

Those days are gone, to be sure, but don't focus too much on the things you have lost. Open yourself to this new feeling overwhelming you. It can feel good to be brimming with something so great and so unexplainable. When the resentment comes, sigh, take a deep breath and gaze at your newborn's face. Really look. See the shape of the eyebrows, the curve of the rosebud lips, the way their eyelashes lay against their cheeks while sleeping. You have given everything and given up everything, but your salvation lies before you. When you find yourself in need of encouragement, gaze at your baby. As you watch, your anger will ebb; and the embers of your love will rekindle. Soon, the love will fill you again and you will remember why you are up for the third night in a row, exhausted, rocking your baby because his tummy hurts.

chapter 27

Babies Don't Keep

Mothering is a challenging task, yet it can be done in a way that is healthy and good for both of you. Your baby will demand the world, and then some, and you, with your love, will try to give it. But an empty pot pours no tea. Without taking care of yourself, how are you going to care for another? This is an often-misunderstood fact about motherhood. We love our babies so much we would walk backwards through fire for them, yet we do not realize we are as much in need of our care as our newborns.

For the first six weeks after a baby is born, you should consider yourself like a baby as well. You are as innocent and new to this thing of motherhood as the baby is to its surroundings. This is true even if this is not your first baby. Each new baby births a new mother. In this new and fragile state, you are as much in need of quiet and rest as your baby.

During the first six weeks, try not to resume any of your previous responsibilities, if possible. If you were working before the birth, try to schedule as much maternity leave as you can get, at least six weeks. If there are other children in your home, arrange before the birth to have help in caring for them once the baby is born. Enlist outside help for housekeeping and cooking duties. Friends and family can drop off ready-made dinners and can come to play with the baby, giving you a break. Or they can take older children with them to give you and the baby some quiet time.

There are countless unforeseen challenges you will face during the postpartum period, when so much is happening as the baby adjusts to being its own person and you adjust to being yourself again. By taking care of what you can foresee (organizing care for your other children, getting help with the housework), you free yourself to face other challenges without having to worry about so many things. Eventually you will have to pick up the reins and get the "team" moving again as mother of the household, but don't expect that of yourself right away.

Rest is essential after birth, so rest as much as you can. Coast through this time. Do only what you have to. One of the biggest challenges of having a new baby will be lack of sleep. If you were used to deep, unbroken sleep (except for occasional trips to the bathroom), this new role as a mother is liable to shock you. I lived in a fog for the first six months postpartum.

My first baby was a good baby; he rarely cried; he was sweet and quiet; but he was also big at birth and really big at two weeks. He nursed every two hours around the clock for five months. That didn't leave me much sleeping time. The first time he slept for five hours straight, I awoke with a start, my mind clear for the first time in forever and there he was, just beginning to stir and famished from his long nursing fast. I snuggled him next to me to nurse, and we both fell back to sleep. The next day, I felt better than I had since he had been born. Those few extra hours of sleep made a big difference.

The exhaustion that comes from getting only broken sleep is not inevitable, however. There are a couple of good ways to prevent feeling so tired all of the time. One simple rule to follow that will help you recover from the birth as well as help with sleep deprivation is to make a habit of resting each time your baby sleeps during the day. Sleep yourself, if you can; if not, lie down and be quiet. Your baby will sleep for nearly twenty-two out of every twenty-four hours for the first few days. Use this time to rest. Nature allowed this time as a recovery and adjustment period for new mothers. Taking advantage of it will keep exhaustion at bay.

Another technique for keeping well-rested is to practice the deep relaxation exercise from the prenatal yoga class that you did during the pregnancy in anticipation of the birth. If you omit the visualization that is part of the prenatal class, you have a traditional version of this exercise. The deep quality relaxation and rejuvenation you feel from doing this exercise, which you may remember from your pregnancy, makes it very beneficial for the postpartum period.

One more thing to remember while trying to coast through these trying first six weeks is that your baby is little for only a short time. This is such a special time that you only get to experience with your child once, so don't waste it by thinking you should be doing something else. Do your baby now; everything else can wait.

My mother gave me a plaque when my first baby was born:

Cleaning and scrubbing can wait till tomorrow,
For babies grow up, we have learned to our sorrow.
So, quiet down cobwebs, and dust go to sleep,
I am rocking my baby and babies don't keep.

Try to remember this when your dishes are stacked to the ceiling right next to the laundry that has taken over the hallway. Try to remember this when you're trying to decide how much time to take before you pick up your responsibilities on the work front.

This is definitely a challenging time, but it is also one of great wonder. If ever there was a time to stop and smell the proverbial roses, this is it.

chapter 28

Mama Juice

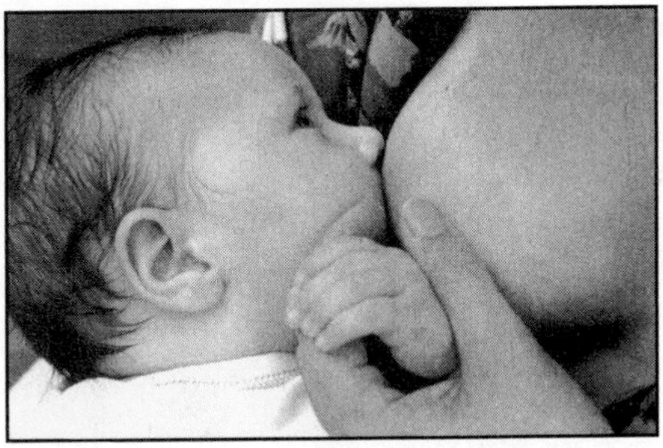

Watching a baby suckling, you can feel the contentment. Babies love to nurse. Nothing is better to a newborn than suckling its mother's breast. As her mother, you were all she knew of the world while *in utero.* Now, having you as the source of food, as well as of love and care, your baby seems to experience a continuation of the deep bond she felt while in the womb. Cradled in your arms, her eyes closing in contentment as warm milk fills her belly, she never seems happier than when she is at the breast.

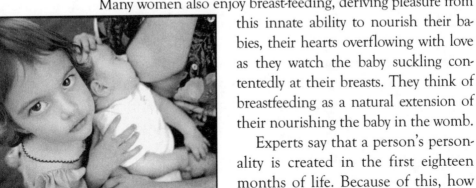

Many women also enjoy breast-feeding, deriving pleasure from this innate ability to nourish their babies, their hearts overflowing with love as they watch the baby suckling contentedly at their breasts. They think of breastfeeding as a natural extension of their nourishing the baby in the womb.

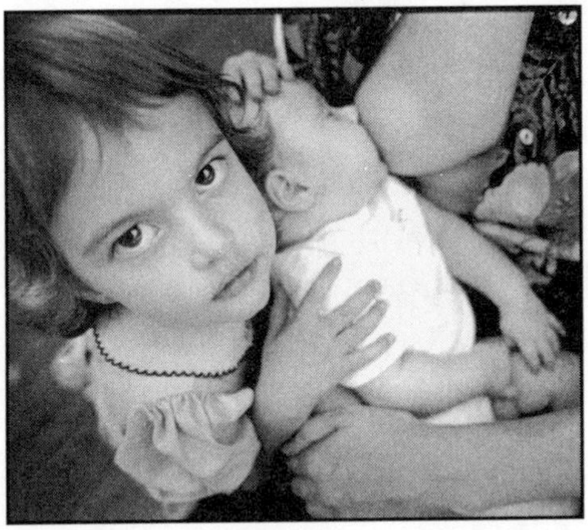

Experts say that a person's personality is created in the first eighteen months of life. Because of this, how your child views the world and self is directly linked to what kind of care they receive as an infant and toddler.

When you come into physical contact with your baby, as you do during breastfeeding, you are giving your child a specific kind of care. The touch of your skin, the closeness of your body, and the attention you shower on your baby while it suckles at the breast is like the light of the Sun to your newborn. Shining on them, it nourishes them and helps them to grow. While feeding your baby, you can feel that exchange of energy passing from you to your baby and back again. The bond that was created between you in the womb is still strong and can be easily felt as you hold your baby in your arms, pouring love and attention onto him. Babies feel this kind of energy easily. They are so new and open to this world that they have not yet learned how to block out the energy of others. This is why babies often fret and cry when there is nothing apparently wrong with them. And this is why they often nurse as much for enjoyment as for nourishment.

Because of this mutual pleasure often experienced by both mother and baby, breastfeeding can be wonderful and fulfilling. However, like everything else having to do with children, it can also be challenging and difficult.

The first couple days after birth your breasts do not produce milk at all. They produce a special substance called colostrum, often called the "first milk." In hospitals, this milk is usually expressed from the breast and discarded, and the infant is fed sugar water until the true milk comes in. First milk is very important for the new baby as it is vitamin rich, with a high protein content, and full of the mother's antibodies to be passed onto the newborn whose undeveloped immune system has no way yet of fighting off disease. To discard this very important first milk is knowingly putting the baby at risk.

Each time you sit down to breastfeed, you will have a "let-down" effect. As your baby latches onto the nipple, hormones are released into your bloodstream sending a signal to your breasts to produce milk. A few moments later, the milk "comes-in" allowing the baby to drink until satisfied.

About seventy-two hours after the baby is born, your "regular" milk will begin to be produced. With only colostrum in your breasts, they may still resemble the breasts you had before pregnancy. When around the third day after the birth, the milk comes in, your breasts become so full of milk, they look huge, even ridiculous. My first experience of breast engorgement had my baby nursing from a breast that was larger than his head! He didn't seem to mind. Fat and happy, he soaked up the milk.

Along with the arrival of your "regular" milk, comes one of the first challenges of breastfeeding: engorgement. Characterized by the full-to-bursting effect that occurs as the milk comes into your breasts for the first time, all at once, some women find engorgement painful; others find it disconcerting, but have no pain. If you have pain, take a warm shower or bath to ease the discomfort. Loosely binding your breasts with a soft cotton cloth to give them support, but without the restrictions of a bra, may also help.

Don't be surprised if it seems that as much milk as the baby drinks, the same amount seems to pour freely from your breast, soaking everything in sight. This is nature's overflow mechanism and will help you feel better.

During engorgement, your breasts learn how much milk they need to produce based upon your baby's nursing patterns. The more your baby suckles, the more milk your breasts will produce. This is why the recommendation to "Feed only on schedule, every four hours, to prevent the baby from being demanding," can result in a failure in breast-feeding. The baby should be demanding as this "demand" is what produces the milk.

It has always fascinated me that my breasts know how much food my baby needs. The baby nurses and if there isn't enough milk, he nurses more. Twenty-four hours later, my breasts will meet the new demands and produce enough milk to keep him full and happy. He determines by his nursing how much he needs and "speaks" to my breasts, commanding more. Without my direct involvement, my breasts comply.

Meanwhile, I'm starving and constantly thirsty as my body searches for the nutrients to replenish itself.

The initial engorgement period lasts two or three days while your body gets used to how much milk is needed. Later you may have minor repeat versions of the initial effect.

When engorgement happens, occasionally all of the milk is not drained from the breast and a clogged or blocked milk duct occurs. Felt as a very sore spot or painful lump in the soft tissue of your breast, blocked ducts occur much more frequently when outside influences are present. Exhaustion or trauma to the soft glandular tissue of the breast are two such influences. Wearing a bra that fits too snugly also seems to precipitate a blocked duct, as the restrictive nature of the device doesn't allow for the proper flow of milk.

When you have a blocked duct, try to make sure that all of the milk is drained from the breast with the blockage. It can also help to gently massage the sore spot, rubbing toward the nipple as the baby nurses. While ducts can be painful, they generally go away on their own unless they progress into mastitis, which is infection of the breast. This condition produces a red, very painful breast and is often accompanied by a fever. If you suspect you have mastitis, you should contact your practitioner.

Another difficulty that can accompany the initial engorgement is the so-called "baby blues." Disconcerting though they are, baby blues are normal. Some women never experience them at all, some only to a little degree, and some find them crippling.

I wept through my first experience of baby blues, wondering how I could be so unhappy with the most perfect person in the world lying on my lap. They hit me at two in the afternoon, three days after Sampath was born, as I sat with him sleeping on my lap. My rear end was still sore from the birth; my neck had a crick from looking at him so much; and my breasts were the size of footballs. All at once, it was all too much and the tears came fast and freely. I knew the blues were the result of powerful hormone changes in my system, but even so, trying to keep my emotional balance was like surfing in high waves. I felt insecure, unable to cope. I was solely responsible for the health of another person, my body hurt, I was tired and hungry all the time—how was I ever going to survive motherhood?

From that experience I learned that the blues are most often short-lived. They come, and they go, and all I had to do was be willing to go through them.

However the blues present themselves to you, try to recognize them for what they are and treat yourself gently. Now is not the time to be thinking about getting up to vacuum the living room or rearrange the closets. When the blues come, just be blue. Cry, lament, whine. Go to bed with your baby and stay there. Let everyone else take care of things for a while. The feeling of being overwhelmed is only a temporary one. Six weeks later, you will feel differently. Honor this process and don't try to fight it and the blues will leave you soon enough.

Differing from the baby blues is postpartum depression. This serious hormonal imbalance can make you feel tired and sad all of the time. Alternately, it can make you feel irritable and angry. If you find that you aren't able to cope on a daily basis, or if you are tired and depressed without a reason such as sleep deprivation, you should contact your practitioner to have them check for post-partum depression.

Another complication to breastfeeding is nipple soreness or cracking. The soft tissue of the nipple, being unused to the suckling of the baby, may become very tender from the unfamiliar pulling action. To help prevent this from happening, prepare in advance by exposing your breasts as often as you can to fresh air and sunshine. This will help toughen the skin somewhat in preparation for nursing.

A cracked nipple, which is extremely painful, can result when the baby does not latch onto the nipple properly. By sucking on only part of it, the strong pulling action causes the skin on one side of the nipple to be pulled very hard and possibly to tear. To prevent this, when your baby nurses, make sure he takes the entire nipple into his mouth.

If you get a tear, put lanolin on it or, even better, petroleum-based calendula ointment, which can be found at your local health food store or a pharmacy which carries homeopathic remedies. Put this cream on immediately after the baby has nursed, seeing that the nipple is dry first. When it is time for the baby to nurse again, make sure that you wipe the cream off before nursing. Nipple soreness without a tear or laceration of the skin will last only a few days; a tear can last for a week or ten days. Be sure to continue nursing even though your nipples are sore. Your nipple will be most sore when the baby first latches on, the pain will lessen after that as the baby suckles.

Most of these problems occur within the first four weeks. Usually by six weeks post-partum, most of the kinks have been ironed out and breastfeeding becomes the enjoyable and fulfilling experience it was meant to be. It is helpful during the early adjustment period for you to have someone around who has breastfed before who can help you through any difficulties. If no one you know has breastfed her baby, check out La Leche League. An international organization dedicated to supporting women in their choice to breastfeed, La Leche League has a wealth of information available to help you with breastfeeding concerns. Their website is www.lalecheleague.org (phone: 847-519-775).

chapter 29

Bed Habits

Once the baby is born the inevitable question comes of where the baby should sleep. These days, it is commonly recommended that the baby sleep separate from the parents, either in the same room, or in another room altogether. As with so many baby-rearing practices, I cannot understand this.

Nearly every woman on leaving her sleeping child will look down into the cradle and long to take her baby into her arms and carry it to the bed to lie snuggled against her breast. Nearly every woman will awaken many times in the night to check on her infant and she will either fight the urge by lying awake and worrying in bed or she will pad a dozen times down the hall to the nursery to make sure the baby is all right. We cannot help doing this. Nature created us perfectly, and perfect mothering means total protection and caring for our young. One of the ways we show this caring is by checking on our babies in the middle of the night to insure that they are safe, warm, and content.

Having a baby in bed next to you can make this kind of caring easier. With the baby there in your bed, you can wake and check on the baby simply by reaching out. If you breastfeed, you have the convenience of nursing the little one without ever having to get out of bed. Snuggled next to your warm body, a baby cared for like this rarely cries. When they wake up, they squirm and make hungry baby noises. With the baby in such close proximity, this alone is enough to wake you.

Before they have a reason to wail, you will be right there, able to talk to them, pull them close, offer your breast, or scoop them up to go get a bottle, and make them safe and secure again. Suckling, they drift right back to sleep.

For natural mothering, sleeping the baby in the parents' bed makes sense. Not only convenient from the mother's point of view, this arrangement is also preferable from the point of view of the baby. After nine months of knowing only you, having you close is what makes your baby feel happiest. Sleeping close to your warmth, listening to the lulling sound of your rythymic breathing as they sleep, hearing your voice so close when they awaken, all add to making the baby feel safe and secure. From this kind of closeness, they get a sense that you are always there for them whenever they need you.

Occasionally fathers object to having a baby in the bed. One of the reasons for this is a fear for the baby's safety. Their babies are so little that many fathers fear that they will roll over in the middle of the night and crush the infant. Relax, fathers: this doesn't happen. Women are not the only beings created perfectly; you also were designed with the particular ability to care for your offspring, and rolling over them in the middle of the night is not part of the design. If you don't believe me, ask other fathers who have slept with their babies. They will tell you that despite some misgivings, they were immediately aware of their babies in the bed next to them even while they slept. And after a few days adjustment period where you might not sleep well because of the fear of rolling over on the baby, you could find that you enjoy having your baby in bed where you can hug and snuggle them whenever you like.

There are a couple of things you need to be concerned with if you sleep the baby in bed with you. Being aware of these things will allow you to take a few precautions to help insure the baby's safety in the expanse of your bed. One concern is of the baby falling out of the bed. A good way to prevent this is for the mother to sleep on the side of the bed that is next to the wall. The wall acts as a barrier to prevent the baby from rolling out. If you do this, line the crack between the bed and the wall with a blanket to prevent the baby from falling down in between the bed and the wall. If your bed is in the middle of the room, you may place a pillow on the edge of the bed to prevent the baby from rolling off. There are also barricades specifically for this purpose. You can find one anywhere that sells baby accessories. At the top of your bed, place another rolled up blanket against the headboard or the wall. This will prevent the baby from falling into that opening.

A second concern is of the baby being covered by your blankets. Prevent this by sleeping the baby higher than the top of the cover and give the baby its own blanket to insure its warmth.

No matter where you sleep your baby, it is usually recommended to sleep your baby on its back or side during the early part of its life. This is because the baby's neck will not be strong enough to hold its head up for quite a while. A baby slept on its stomach could literally smother from not being able to lift its head up to breathe. Sleeping a baby on its back is a better choice, as a baby will breathe easily in this position, but it does carry some risk as the baby could choke if it were to spit up while on its back.

Sleeping the baby on its side will allow it to be able to breathe easily and will reduce the risk of its choking. While your baby is very young, you will need to place something behind its back to prevent it from rolling over during sleep. This can be accomplished by taking a rolled up cotton receiving blanket and laying it snugly against its back. As your baby grows, and is able to hold up its head and sit on its own, sleeping position is no longer a concern.

chapter 30

Massage Message

Massaging a newborn is one of the most enjoyable and fulfilling activities you can participate in. As parents, we long to touch our newborns from the moment of their births. We want to go over every finger, every limb, marveling at the wonder we've created. Massage gives us the opportunity to do this, while being very nice for the baby, as well.

A wonderful massage you can do from the very first day your

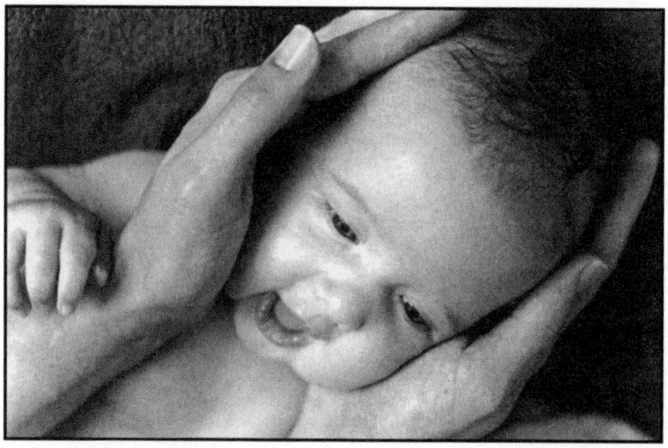

baby is born is a castor oil massage. A time-honored East Indian tradition reputed to reduce the heat in the baby's system caused by the friction of birth, it also makes the baby's skin lovely and soft, even on wrinkly feet. Buy your castor oil from a local health food store, or pharmacy and try to get "cold-pressed" if you can. If you are unable to locate it locally, it can be ordered through the mail from The Heritage Store (P.O. Box 444-WWW, Virginia Beach, VA, 23458; phone 1-800-862-2923; or online at www.caycecures.com).

In preparation for the massage, make sure your room is nice and warm. Lay a towel on the bed or the floor and lay a receiving blanket over it to make a nice, soft place for the baby

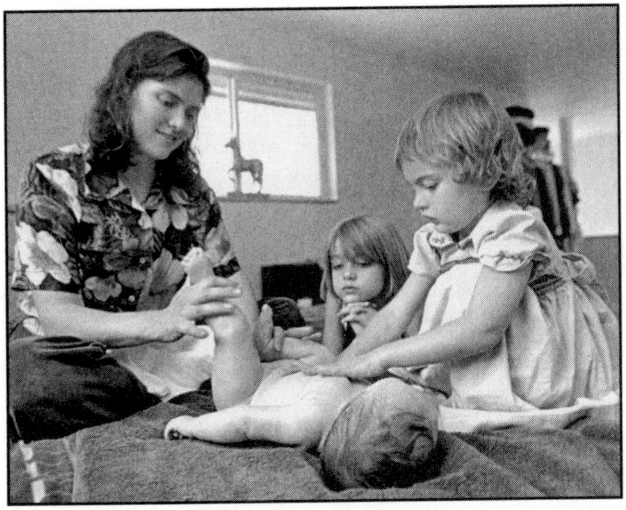

to lie. You may also want to place a sheet of plastic beneath the towel in case the baby pees while you are in the middle of the massage. Have another blanket or two close by to cover the parts of the baby you are not massaging to keep the baby warm. If it is the middle of summer, or you are in a very hot room, this may not be necessary.

Warm your hands by rubbing them together, or running them under hot water. Undress your baby and lay her face up on the towel. Pour about a tablespoon of oil into your palms and rub them together to warm the oil. Beginning with the chest area, slowly and gently rub the oil onto the baby, starting from the center and moving down to the sides. You will notice the oil is very sticky. Rub the oil onto the baby very slowly so you don't pull the skin, adding more oil to keep your hands well lubricated.

After the chest, move to the abdomen and rub in small circles, clockwise in the direction the large intestines move. If your baby has not had a first bowel movement, expelling the sticky, brownish-black meconium that filled the intestines while the baby was *in utero,* don't be surprised if the castor oil massage stimulates this expulsion.

After the abdomen, move to the legs. Gently massage from the feet toward the hips, which helps to return the blood from the legs to the heart, and then massage the feet themselves. Rubbing in little circles in the center of the feet and on the heel for the accupressure points for the colon can also help to stimulate the expulsion of the meconium. From the feet move to the arms and massage from the wrists to the shoulders, and then the hands, gently rubbing the palm to stimulate the colon.

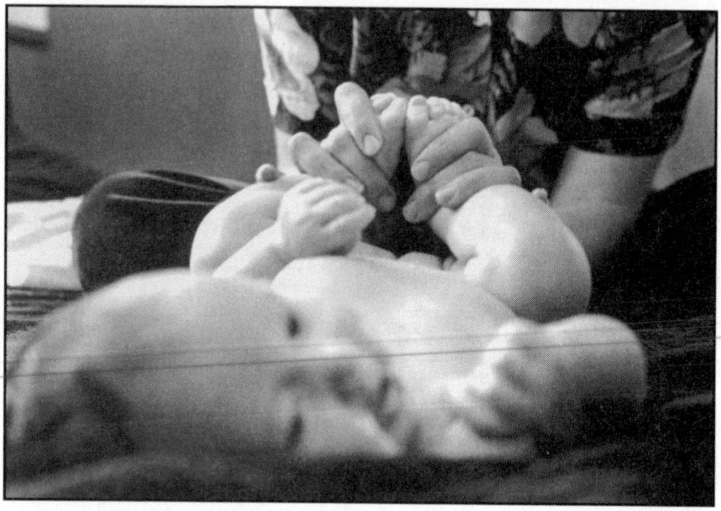

Next, carefully roll the baby over and massage the back, stroking from the center out to the sides. Rub up in around the neck and down all over the buttocks. Last, roll the baby back over and massage the face and head. It is fine to get the oil in the baby's hair and ears, just remember to be careful with the soft spot on the top of the baby's head where the bones have not yet closed.

After you are done, wrap the baby in a receiving blanket, and another warm blanket and, if it is at all cold, put a hat on the baby's head. The baby will seem very sticky for about twelve hours until all of the castor oil has been absorbed. Then you will notice that any dry skin is gone, and that everything, including the hair, is soft and silky.

You can give your baby a castor oil bath as often as you like, even every day is not too frequently and for as long as you like, as they never seem to outgrow their love of massage. Whenever I start to massage one of my children, the others line up and the next thing I know, there are five sets of feet to work on and five bare backs that want to be stroked. Fortunately, I have never outgrown that longing to touch them either.

chapter 31

The Lifelong Challenge

The lights over the stove are making me hot. I wrinkle my forehead in exasperation; I don't seem to be able to cut the broccoli fast enough. I set the broccoli down and pick up the pasta pot. Carrying it to the sink, I trip over a pan lid.

"Damn it! Who put that there?" Not waiting for a reply I kick it out of my way and shove the pot in the sink. Turning the water on, I tap my fingers on the edge of the sink anxiously waiting while the pot fills. Dinner is going to be late again, I sigh, noticing the band of tension that has settled across my forehead. I'm tired and stressed from the events of the day and dinner is going to be late, again.

The pot is full. I grab it.

"Mama?"

"What?" I answer, irritably, not looking, not turning around.

"Mama?" it comes again.

"I said 'what' already. Now, what do you want?"

I put the pan on the stove, turn the burner on beneath it, and go back to the broccoli. "Mama?"

I try a different tack.

"Not, now, Mama's trying to get dinner ready."

"Maamaa?!?"

"Not now!" I shout.

Silence behind me.

I stop. I inhale deeply and let it out slowly through my mouth. I notice the steam rising off the water, awaiting the pasta, steam rising up and dissipating into the kitchen air. I take another breath, in, out. I notice how green the broccoli is against the white cutting board, how shiny the knife is. I lay the knife down. I turn around.

On the floor my eight-month-old baby, Lalita, has made a drum set with my pots and pans, having pulled them out from under the sink. She looks at me looking down at her and grins, showing her two teeth. She's so cute, I give a half grin back. That small smile eases some of the tension on my forehead.

From under the table three-year-old Madhuri looks up at me.

"Mama?" she says, again, now that I am looking at her.

"What?" I ask her, softer now.

"I love you." She says, giggling, her cheeks dimpling.

Oh, dear.

"Come here, Sweetie." I say, bending down as she scampers over to give me a hug.

"I love you, too. Very much."

She smiles and kisses me on both cheeks before returning to her hideaway under the table. Twelve-year-old Sampath, gets up from the table and walks over.

He mock-scowls at the baby, and makes a grab for Madhuri as she peeks from under the table. Then he turns to me, "Mom, check it out." He shows me the picture in a Nintendo 64 game catalog of a game he'd like to get called "Monster Truck Madness." "Cool, huh?"

"I guess so." I reply, ruffling his hair as he grins at me hopefully. Suddenly the need to get dinner done doesn't seem quite so urgent.

I turn slowly and grab another head of broccoli off the counter. Carrying it to the kitchen sink I step over the drum set. The baby chortles. Outside my kitchen window my other son, Nataraja, the ten-year-old daredevil, races his bike across the yard. He sees me watching and deliberately wipes out. I flinch. He gets up unhurt and dusts himself off, looking at me expectantly.

"I don't really get hurt," he told me last week, "I just like to crash because it gets me more attention." I'm not sure I like his reasoning, but I give him two thumbs up and a mock applause, anyway. He grins, delighted, picks up his bike and heads to the top of the yard to do it again.

On the trampoline at the top of the garden, my eldest daughter, six-year-old Rani, dances and twirls, and waves when she sees me watching. With her hair and her dress bouncing in opposition to the rest of her, she looks so funny I have to laugh. I wave back. The broccoli washed, I take it back to the counter and cut it slowly.

The water is boiling, ready for the pasta. I pour it in, a few at a time, watching it slide beneath the water. In a few minutes, this pasta, inedible now, will be soft and pliable, ready to nourish us. Without boiling, it would be good for nothing.

I think about that. I am like that pasta. Hard and cold, I am good to no one. But if I let myself remember and be warmed by the love surrounding me, if I shed my "package of the day," the worries and cares that have cloaked me, and allow myself to be transformed by what is happening now, then I, too will become soft, able to nourish my children. I sigh and relax, the anxiousness has gone.

"Mama?" I hear again. I stop and turn around.

"Yes, little lady?" I say to Madhuri.

"I love you."

"I know, Cutie-pie, I love you too."

So many evenings are stressful for me. Sometimes preparing a meal at the end of a long work-day takes more energy than I think I have left. Into that weary exhaustion, my children act as a reminder, showing me again and again what is really important. They show me that every moment is precious, and every moment holds the potential for joy.

So, dinner is late again. Make it thirty seconds later. Take that time to stop and be with your child. Sometimes the only thing a child wants is thirty seconds in which to share a smile. Stop and share it with them. What our children really want from us is our time and attention, our love and appreciation. They want to share with us all that they see as wonderful *today*: a new game in a magazine, a song they learned at school, a story from their lives. Don't waste this time with them getting wrapped up in all of the work that comes with caring for children and missing the little things that make having children the joy it is.

You will face so many challenges raising your children: scraped knees, bloody noses, nightmares, wet beds, arguments, crying fits; everything you are and everything you know will be tasked by this process of creating the next generation. In the midst of this chaos, learn to stop and take the time to be there with them as they grow. Don't let a day go by without hugging them and telling them that you love them. It is a wonderful journey that began with the birth of your baby. It will allow you to sit back and rediscover the world through a new pair of eyes. Don't lose the magic of this experience by being caught up in the physical demands of raising children. Remember every day what a gift it is to be alive and to have been able to give life to another.

Remember that birth, as a gift, was not meant to be scary. It was meant to test you, to prepare you for this greater journey of caring for your young. It was meant as an exercise in honoring yourself and in learning to depend on your inner strength. It was meant to make you feel more powerful and more capable than you were before the experience.

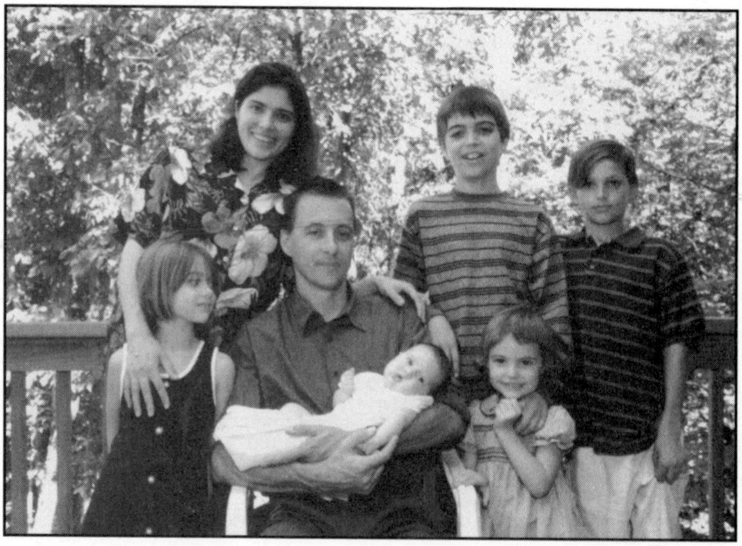

Left to right in a clockwise circle: Rani, Lakshmi, Sampath, Nataraja, Madhuri, Nilakantan and Lalita in center.

Resources

Waterbirth Resources

Author's Website
e-mail: info@choosingwaterbirth.com
website: www.choosingwaterbirth.com
Contains resources, information, and stories on water birth and natural birth.

Active Birth Centre
Janet Balaskas
25 Bickerton Road
London
N19 5JT
UK
Phone: + 44 (0) 171-482-5554
Fax: + 44 (0) 171-267-9683
e-mail: info@activebirthcentre.com
website: www.activebirthcentre.com

The Active Birth Centre offers informative education to help with the emotional and physical preparation for birth and early parenting designed to empower and inspire women to have confidence in their ability to give birth and to aid them in choosing the right birth option for their particular circumstances. Provides information on waterbirth, prenatal yoga, and aromatherapy.

Aquadoula
PO Box 1132
110 9th Av. S.
Edmonds, WA 98020
Phone: 1-888-217-2229
Fax: (425) 776-2157

e-mail: waterbirth@aquadoula.com
website: www.aquadoula.com

Provider of portable spas designed specifically for water labor and delivery. The spas are soft, yet sturdy, easy to set up, and lightweight and compact for easy shipping. Pricing and rental information available online.

Birth Balance
Judith Elaine Halek, Director
309 W. 109th St. Apt. 6D
New York, NY 10025
Phone: (212) 222-4349
Fax: (212) 222-8308
Birth Balance is the east coast resource center for underwater birth providing support and information including video and photo documentation of the International Waterbirth Conferences, a resource list of centers and practitioners offering waterbirth, and a newsletter.

Birth Center of the Blue Ridge
1380 East Rio Road
Charlottesville, VA 22901
Phone: (804) 977-4757
Fax: (804) 977-0411

Provides safe, sensitive, and specialized care in a warm and friendly, home-like environment for women choosing to experience natural births and waterbirths in Central Virginia. The birth center I chose when I gave birth to my fifth baby, Lalita Karensa.

Point of View Productions and The Waterbirth Website
Karil Daniels
2477 Folsom St.
San Francisco, CA 94110
Phone: (415) 821-0435
website: www.well.com/user/karil

Producer/Director of *WATER BABY: Experiences of WaterBirth*, award winning documentary that features four waterbirths and the world's top waterbirth pioneer doctors, and home of "The Waterbirth Website" providing a wealth of information about waterbirth including an extensive waterbirth resource list to help you locate a practitioner in your area.

Waterbirth International
Global Maternal/Child Health Association
Barbara Harper
PO Box 1400
Wilsonville, OR 97070
Phone: (503) 682-3600
e-mail: waterbirth@aol.com
website: www.waterbirth.org

The Global Maternal/Child Health Association and Waterbirth International Research, Resource, and Referral Service is a non-profit organization dedicated to assisting women and their families discover the benefit of laboring and giving birth in water. The website has a waterbirth store, a frequently asked questions section, information on locating portable pools, and a referral service to aid in locating a practitioner.

Natural Birth and Midwifery Resources:

The American College of Nurse Midwives (ACNM)
818 Connecticut Ave. NW, Suite 900
Washington, DC 20006
Phone: (202) 728-9860
Fax: (202) 728-9897
E-mail: info@acnm.org
Website: www.acnm.org

Providing research, accreditation for nurse-midwifery programs; administers and promotes continuing education programs; establishes clinical practice standards; and creates liaisons with state, and federal agencies and members of Congress.

International Childbirth Education Association (ICEA)
PO Box 20048
Minneappolis, MN 55420
Phone: (952) 854-8600
Fax: (952) 854-8772
e-mail: info@icea.org
website: www.icea.org

Offers professional certification programs, childbirth educator workshops, and an annual international convention. Website provides a bookstore, a membership roster of over 8,000 members, certification and childbirth education information for those interested in childbirth educators, Doulas, and labor support people.

Lamaze International
1200 19th Street, NW, Suite 300
Washington, DC 20036-2422
Phone: 1-800-368-4404
Fax: (202) 429-5112
e-mail: lamaze@cd.sba.com
website: lamaze-childbirth.com

Through education, advocacy, and reform, Lamaze International seeks to promote normal, natural, healthy, and fulfilling childbearing experiences for women and their families. Website has a bookstore and media center and information for childbirth educators, health care providers, and parents-to-be.

Magazines:

Birth Gazette

42 The Farm
Summertown, TN 38483-9626
Phone: (931) 964-3798
e-mail: brthgzt@usit.net
www.birthgazette.com

A quarterly magazine published by Pamela Hunt and Ina May Gaskin, author of the best-selling *Spiritual Midwifery*, concerning midwifery, childbirth, and the politics of health care.

The Compleat Mother

PO Box 209
Minot, ND 58702
Phone: (701) 852-2822
e-mail: greg@rsq.org
website: www.compleatmother.com

A quarterly magazine of pregnancy, birth, and breastfeeding for the purpose of promoting natural, enjoyable birth and extended breastfeeding.

Midwifery Today

PO Box 2672-350
Eugene, OR 97402
Phone: (541) 344-7438
e-mail: inquiries@midwiferytoday.com
website: www.midwiferytoday.com

A quarterly journal about pregnancy, labor, and birth for midwives, nurses, doulas, childbirth educators and practitioners, and parents-to-be.

Mothering

PO Box 1690
Santa Fe, NM 87504
Phone: (505) 984-8116
e-mail: info@mothering.com
website: www.mothering.com

The natural family living magazine released monthly containing information on birth and pregnancy, motherhood, and child rearing.

Nurturing Magazine
#373,918-16th Ave. NW
Calgary
Alberta Canada
T2M OK3
e-mail: webmistress@nurturing.com
website: www.nurturing.com

A monthly magazine whose primary goal is the discussion of the importance of the family unit and child raising with articles on home schooling, breastfeeding, home birth, and more.

About the Author

In writing about waterbithing for prospective parents, Lakshmi Bertram found a way to combine her two passions—mothering and yoga—in one helpful expression. A mother of five and a student of yoga for years, Lakshmi lives in central Virginia with the Yogaville spiritual community, founded by Sri Swami Satchidananda, who also developed the style of hatha yoga known as Integral Yoga. Lakshmi frequently lectures on the benefits of yoga during pregnancy and natural birthing techniques, and continues to write about childrearing and motherhood.

Author's Note About the Photographer

All of the pictures in this book were taken by one very talented photographer: Stephanie Gross. She posesses the skill, talent, and the "eye" to capture visually the essence of what I wanted to say, and had the added benefit of being unassuming and authentic, making her energy perfect for this project. Working with her was a pleasure in all ways, and I couldn't have been more pleased with what she brought to this book through her photographs.

Stephanie is a freelance photographer. She lives on a farm in the foothills of the Blue Ridge Mountains with her husband Charles, two cats, and four dogs. She has a BFA in photography from the Rhode Island School of Design, and spent ten years as a newspaper photographer. Her pictures have appeared in the *Washington Post*, the *New York Times*, and *Glamour Magazine*. You may contact Stephanie through e-mail at stephphoto@hotmail.com. Or you may write to her at 795 Falling Rock Dr., Amherst VA 24521.

Index